AM I DEAD YET?

A story of addiction
and the power of hope

HEATHER GAINES

Am I Dead Yet?
© 2020 Heather Gaines. All rights reserved.

Print ISBN: 978-0-578-73165-0
E-Book ISBN: 978-0-578-73166-7

First Printing: 2020
Printed in the United States of America
10 9 8 7 6 5 4 3 2 1

Credits:
Managing Editor: Jenny Peterson
Content Editing & Design: LeAnn Zotta
Proofreading: Stephen Wilson
Produced by The Garden of Words, LLC
TheGardenOfWords.com

This publication was produced using available information. The publisher regrets it cannot assume responsibility for errors or omissions.

Names, events, places, and conversations were recreated from memory for this book. To maintain the anonymity of the individuals herein, names, places and/or identifying characteristics and details may have been changed. Any resemblance to persons living or dead is purely coincidental.

DEDICATION

This book is dedicated to the still sick and suffering, whether you
are an alcoholic, an addict, or a cancer patient.
There is always HOPE.

TABLE OF CONTENTS

RESTAURANT CAREER

FOREWORD

We all go through tough times in life. Maybe they're of our own doing, maybe they're out of our control. We struggle and struggle, and wonder when life will be better. It happens to all of us at some point.

Heather Gaines has had a life that's been tough from the beginning, coming from a loving family that just had issues. Heather brought those issues with her into her adulthood, and her life got even tougher than anyone could ever imagine. And then, Heather turned it around—she was lucky to have had help and a lot of people who loved and supported her. Not only did she turn it around but she turned it around in a *spectacular* way.

I met Heather 12 years ago when we were both doing these crazy early morning workouts with a retired Navy Chief. Not too many people would put themselves through this type of grueling physical and emotional work, but Heather was on the path of health after she'd dealt with her alcohol and drug addiction. She was there every single morning, never missing a workout, until she was diagnosed with a devastating disease.

Most people would be tempted to give up, to throw in the towel. Most people would think, "After all the work I've done to turn my life around, and this is what happens?" Others would use it as an excuse to go off the wagon and slip back into their old, unhealthy patterns and habits.

Not Heather! She had this amazing attitude that it was just another bump in the road, another blip on the radar. She would do what she needed to do and be back as soon as she could—and when she did come back, she was physically and mentally stronger than ever. She used the experience and growth from her earlier challenges and just applied it to this new one, inspiring everyone around her.

I became Heather's boss when she came to work at my business, Lazy Dog. There she became a SUP (Stand-Up Paddleboard) instructor, a tour guide, and a PaddleFit Instructor. You think a workout on land is hard? Heather leads people through workouts on a paddleboard! Ever since meeting her and getting to know her, I've been inspired by her attitude and the way she embraces life. She takes on every day with kindness, understanding, allowance, and a never-stop-winning "let's go!" attitude.

While Heather was writing this book, I watched her relive some of her most difficult memories. That would be hard for anyone, and while I'm sure it wasn't easy for Heather, she stuck with it and just as always, came out stronger. There's one word that always comes to mind when I think of Heather—that word is HOPE.

Whatever it is you're experiencing in your life, however difficult your life may be, or however impossible you may think it is to have the happy life you want—the fact that you have this book in your hands means you are on the right path. It's easy for people to dispense advice when their lives have been a cakewalk, but when you've lived in the darkness that Heather has and come out the other side? You know she offers words of wisdom that you can trust. You know that she has experienced the despair, shame, guilt, and hopelessness that every addict experiences, and yet she is here today as a beautiful and inspiring example of the power of hope.

And even if you're not an addict, and you've never rolled your car down a cliff, done blow with famous musicians, awakened in a crack den, or been diagnosed with cancer, *Am I Dead Yet?* will inspire you to be better, to do better, and to be happier. All it takes is one step towards hope, with Heather as your guide. Just when you think you've had enough and you're ready to give in (or give up), Heather reminds you that you've still got 40% left.

So congratulations! You've picked up this book and are about to embark on the rollercoaster of Heather's life—and just like with actual theme-park rollercoasters, you'll be thrilled, you'll wonder if anyone will make it out alive, you'll laugh, maybe shiver, and then you'll land safely. And even though the ride might be terrifying at times, you'll know that in the end, all is well.

Heather's adventures continue today but this time it's all about the best that life has to offer—grace, hope, love, and possibility.

Now let's go!

Sue Cooper
Owner, Lazy Dog
Heather's friend and boss

PREFACE

I don't know when it came to me, but for a long time, I've wanted to write a book. I have not one story to tell but several. I feel like I'm the equivalent of Peter Pan, a cat with nine lives, a phoenix rising from the ashes, and a girl on a train. (Just kidding, that's already taken.)

Who falls down a flight of stairs, fractures their skull, and lives to tell about it? Who does blow with one of the most famous rock musicians on the planet and can even remember it? Who was just about homeless, living in a hotel full of rats? Who has the most amazing group of people in her life? The answer is little ol' me, and I'm still here. Life experiences are what mold you into who you are.

My life has been a succession of good, bad, funny, sad, crazy...millions of moments and experiences. I consider myself extremely fortunate to be able to share these experiences, especially the hard, uncomfortable ones. If I can give anyone even a chance at hope, a laugh, some tools, a way not sweat the small stuff, then I consider myself a success.

Growing up in California, I thought I had a pretty normal life—that is, until I think back on it. Little glimpses of things that just weren't right, or shouldn't have happened, or did happen and shouldn't have. I didn't really realize the damage done until way later. Dad was an alcoholic, and Mom was probably more co-dependent on Dad than he was on alcohol. Despite all of that, there was a ton of love in my family, as chaotic and crazy as it was.

I was introduced to alcohol at a very early age—eight, I think. I remember my first drink. It was at a New Year's Eve party at a neighbor's house down the street. My little friend and I were there in our pajamas, and I remember a man giving us each a Tequila Sunrise, and I thought it was the most beautiful drink I'd ever seen. The yellow, the orange, the red... it was so beautiful, and just that glistening of the condensation on the outside of the glass... and I remember tasting it and thinking, Oh, this is the greatest thing ever!

My dad used to drink beer. Coors. He always used to give me sips, and that was nice. He would give me sips of his liquor every once in a while, too. It's weird, but it was something we shared. Some people are genetically predisposed to be alcoholic. I don't know if I am or not; most times I think I drank just to be cool. It was cool to sneak around and drink, like my older brothers. I genuinely liked it because it gave me confidence I wouldn't otherwise have had. I also learned that I could drink a lot. I mean a lot. While everybody else was vomiting, I was not. That should have been my first clue.

My life was all about swimming for a long time. Then it was cheerleading. After that, it was drinking, and smoking pot here and there. But most of all, my life was spent trying to fit in, knowing that I didn't. I didn't have everything all the other people had: the nice clothes, the cars, everything I saw that was so shiny and new. I always compared my outsides to other people's outsides and never spent much time trying to figure out the insides.

I don't even remember my mom talking to me about my period. I think she just said, "Hey, here's a pad. This is what happens every month." You know, putting on those pads... holy shit. It was like wearing a goddamn diaper. How could you feel cute or look cute with a fucking big ol' log between your legs?

But that's just, you know, stuff. God bless my mom. She was my hero. She kept a lot of shit together. And I'm amazed that she actually lived as long as she lived. Both my parents passed away in their sixties, and I'm not too far away from that now. I used to think about it when my birthday rolled around, like, Oh, my God, do I only have a few years left? Even my brother died when he was just 49. It does give you pause.

But people say, Heather, you're totally not like your brother or your parents. You're a lot different. You stopped drinking. You don't do drugs. You take care of yourself. You live a life of giving, and work hard at giving hope to others.

You know, those people are right. Now that I've gotten off of Heather's Death-Defying Rollercoaster, my biggest fear is an un-lived life.

Catch you later, and enjoy the book... you might want to buckle up!

———⌁———

Everything was black.

Why do I feel like I've been swimming for forever?

I feel wet. It's dark. I don't know where I'm at. I feel rain dripping on my face.

Was it rain? I struggled to open my eyes, but I couldn't. I didn't know what was happening... was I just dreaming?

Then I felt something on my face. What was that? I tried again to open my eyes... why was it so hard to do? My eyes felt glued shut and I couldn't seem to move my arms.

I finally opened my eyes in the pitch black, and there was a dog licking my face.

I start to see around me a little bit. I was in a house, and there were dogs, just looking at me. I got up and I could not figure out why I was all wet; my head, my shirt?

Where the hell am I?

Am I dead?

PART I
CHILDHOOD

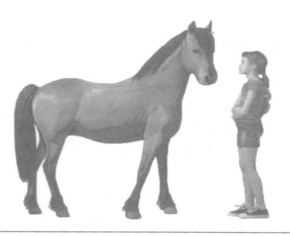

SQUARE ONE

My parents were middle-class people—well, maybe lower-middle class—just ordinary people who lived ordinary suburban lives. My dad was Richard Buford Gaines, a construction worker. My dad's nickname was Dick. Further on down my road in life, that would become pretty appropriate.

My father had a big personality, and reminded me of Frank Sinatra and Bing Crosby back in the day. He had beautiful blue eyes and was six-foot-four, a towering man who was full of charisma and charm. He was also a lethal manipulator who knew how to hide, lie, and cheat to get what he wanted. When I was small, I idolized him. He was the apple of my eye, and I was daddy's little girl.

My mom was Rhoda Louise Gaines. She hated the name Rhoda, so everybody called her Louise. Mom didn't work while her kids were young, and that was the norm in the early '60s. She always packed us a lunch to take to school, and was always home in the afternoon when we came back.

The "us" I'm referring to is my three older brothers and younger sister. I'm Number Four in the order, born in 1961. Richard (also known as "Buff") is the oldest; Chris (also known as "Chris") is second: and Eric (also known as "Dink") is the youngest brother. Elizabeth is my younger sister. We were all born pretty close together, and anyone who remembers can tell you that we were a handful.

Our little house was on a really cool cul-de-sac in a semi-rural California suburb I'll call "Brooktree Hills." There were kids in almost every house who were around the same age as us, so we had built-in playmates. Back in those days, kids were allowed to roam around unsupervised, play in the street, cut through the woods, ride a bike to the store. We didn't care about much more than kickball and tree forts and whether we could get a dime to get something from the ice-cream man. Those things eventually turned into "Spin the Bottle" (and maybe drink what was in it first!). That whole time was about learning to grow up.

The neighbor-kids seemed to have families who had everything. We always seemed to struggle. I think that's because my father was an alcoholic. He wasn't the stereotype of an alcoholic, you know, the man in the trench coat laying in the gutter. He was the man who would go to work and probably drink on the job, but he would try to put food on the table and come home every night. Nowadays they call that a "functioning alcoholic," which is just about the biggest oxymoron I can think of.

We did have one really cool thing, and that was horses: Thunder, a thoroughbred; Jiggs, a Shetland pony; Sherry; an Appaloosa; and Peanuts, a pinto pony. Peanuts was small enough to crawl under the fence and walk into the house if anyone left the door open. Those horses were a big part of my life when I was young—one of the few "normal" things I felt connected to then.

· 2 ·

Not a Good Fit

I don't remember a lot before I was five, so I'll start there. My kindergarten teacher was Mrs. Carlisle, and she was really nice. She even had a kid's show on a local TV channel, so she was kind of famous. On the other hand, my first-grade teacher was really a nasty lady. We used to call her Mrs. Lizard. She's probably still around because she's too mean to die.

Around that time, I discovered that I loved the water and learned to swim. From the age of six, my life was all about swimming. We had a neighborhood swim team and my mom and dad had all of us kids join it. We were all very good at it, but the coaches actually saw some real potential in me. I was swimming, swimming, and swimming some more, and ended up getting private lessons and even a swim coach. In hindsight, I think that probably kept me busy and out of the kind of trouble that first-graders get into. It was about the only place I ever felt I fit in as a young kid.

My second-grade teacher was Mrs. English. Third grade, Mrs. Pumelo. One of my faves was Mrs. Yakamora (fourth grade). She was Japanese and taught us how to eat seaweed, and all about Japanese culture. I have especially nice memories of her class, maybe because she seemed to understand that school was hard for me. I wasn't good at math; I just couldn't get it or concentrate on it because my comprehension was bad. I daydreamed a lot to escape the chaos of living in a home with five young kids that was run by an alcoholic. Eventually, my teachers learned not to sit me near a window because I would just stare at the playground and wish I was somewhere else.

Fifth grade was not fun. In fact, it was awful. My teacher, the extra-horrible Mr. Burlein, was probably a secret alcoholic because we used to see him sneaking things in and out of his locker and drinking mouthwash all the time. He wasn't a very tolerant teacher, so my friend and I always got in trouble—and when we got in trouble, there was always a consequence.

Burlein would say, "OK, Heather, I've asked you to stop talking in class! Now I want you to write 100 times—and turn it in tomorrow—'I will not talk in class!'" That happened more than once. He was very mean to me and made me cry more than once.

I remember the last day of school that year. I stomped up to Mr. Burlein and said,

"You know what, I'm glad I'm not going to see you when I die because you're going to HELL and I'm going to HEAVEN!" And I ran away from him. School was over, so he couldn't suspend me. That meant I was victorious! It was probably the most bold thing I had ever done, because I was brought up to respect my elders and definitely not to talk back.

Mr. Anand, my sixth-grade teacher, was one of my best teachers ever. He *got* me. I could tell him what was happening at home and about the crazy things I did, and he didn't judge me. He made me feel like I could do anything—he gave me encouragement, which I really needed then. I wasn't one of the cute girls and needed all the help I could get.

I may not have been the cutest, but I was definitely one of the *fastest* girls in that elementary school. (The fastest boy was Ben Kiley, and I always had a crush on him.) How could I not be an athletic tomboy with three older brothers?

By the early '70s, the culture had changed a lot and girls didn't have to wear skirts and dresses to school anymore. The fashion trend of the day was Levi's flared hip-hugger jeans. Everyone was wearing them and I really wanted a pair. I begged my mom until she finally caved and said she would buy them for me. I was so excited! She came home one day and announced, "Hooch, I have a surprise for you!" ("Hooch" was my nickname, given to me by my dad. I learned later on that "hooch" is another word for cheap booze. How nice.)

Anyway, I was thinking, *Woohoo, I'm getting jeans!* She pulled the pants out of the bag, all proud of what she picked out. Then, all of my excitement poofed into thin air. *Where are my dark blue hip-hugger bell-bottom Levi's?* These were sky blue, straight-legged, with orange and yellow painter-pant pockets. She was all thrilled to show me what she'd bought, and held them up to my waist to see how they would look. They were way too big.

"No big deal," said Mom. "I'll just take them in." I was so disappointed, but she was so pumped. Money was always tight, and new stuff was usually only for Christmas, so I kept my mouth shut. That Monday, I got dressed for school and put on my too-big brand-new straight-legged jeans. NOTHING was going to stop me from wearing those pants. I put a belt on to keep them from falling down, and went to school. I was very self-conscious, but I wore them with pride.

Too-big jeans = didn't fit in... that's something you'll hear a lot about in this book.

I don't know how I got shaped like that. I just never felt good enough, no matter how hard I tried or how many swimming trophies I won. I got the Presidential Physical Fitness award every single year, and I still didn't feel good enough. That would stay with me for a long, long time.

· 3 ·

Drunk Dad

I always knew when my father was drunk because his eyelids got really droopy and his blue eyes got all watery and extra-blue. Sometimes he'd walk in the house with a scowl on his face, and my mother would just be like, "Not again, Dick." My mom put up with a lot.

I don't know what started my dad drinking, but I remember it getting a lot worse after the Uncle Jim thing.

My dad had a good friend we called Uncle Jim. He wasn't really an uncle, just a good friend of my dad's who was always very nice to me. He was kind of short and stout, and always wore a double-breasted suit that made him look even stouter. Every once in a while he'd coming rolling up in his car to visit. He'd get out of the car and yell, "Hey, Hooch, I got a present for you!" That was an exciting thing for any kid.

He handed me the most awesome stuffed animal, a basset hound. Where this name came from, I don't know, but we called him Axelrod. That stuffed dog went everywhere with me and I had it for years and years. One day I asked my dad whatever happened to Uncle Jim, who hadn't come around for a while.

My dad told me Jim had been on a business trip in San Francisco. He had stopped into a liquor store when a bunch of the Black Panthers came in, held up the store, and killed Uncle Jim. That was really crazy and really, really sad. Just another up-and-down time. Sometimes good things wiped out the bad things, but then bad things would always seem to come back and wipe out the good things.

So much stuff happened behind the scenes that we kids probably didn't know about, but I just knew my mother was very, very unhappy by the time I was nine. I believe I became her sounding board about how Dad was treating her, lying about his drinking, how she couldn't stop him from drinking, how she wanted to leave him, and what should she do? *For Christ's sake!* I was nine years old.

We had this tradition where my dad would take us kids to this deli in town so we could get the ends of the hard salami. The deli couldn't use them for sandwiches and the owner used to just give them to us because my dad knew the owner. It was a special treat because we all loved salami. That little deli was in the same parking lot as the Safeway grocery store.

One day my dad got me and Chris and Dink into the car to go grocery shopping. Dad said, "OK, you guys. Here's your mom's grocery list. Get the stuff on the list and get a fruit rollup for yourselves. I'll stop in the deli and get some sandwich meats." I wanted to go with my dad in hopes of getting a salami-end.

He squirmed a little and said, "No, you go help Chris and Dink in the Safeway. The deli is all out of salami."

I was gullible, but I questioned that. "How can a deli be out of salami?" I asked. "I don't know, Hooch, he's just out," he answered. So I backed off, but something in my head said something was not right.

Like a good little soldier, I followed my brothers over to the Safeway. We went running to the aisle where they kept the fruit rollups. We didn't have a lot of money, so something like a fruit rollup was like a triple-decker ice cream cone to us.

I walked back to the front of the store, watching the deli, waiting for my dad to come out. Chris kept tugging on me to come and help him do the shopping, but I told him to leave me alone. I saw my dad walk out of the deli with a bag in his hand. Then I learned what it meant to see that size of a brown paper bag: it was a pint liquor bottle.

Huh? He told Mom he had stopped drinking.

He walked away from the deli, looking left and right, and walked real fast up to the trunk of our car. He stashed the bag in the trunk and got in the car to wait for us.

I didn't say "mother fucker" back then, but I remember thinking, *What the heck? He's got liquor, but he's not supposed to be drinking.*

Thinking back, that was one of the probably hundreds of times he told my mom he wasn't going to drink. I know he was thinking, *I'll start getting vodka; you can't smell it!* These would be my exact same thoughts years later, ha!

I waited for my brothers to come out of the Safeway and created a diversion by asking them what they got me. I figured if I did that, they wouldn't think I was up to anything. Sneaky Pete, I was.

They had gotten me a cherry rollup. We went and got in the car and my dad said, "Oh, look! I found some salami ends!" My dad was a liar. I knew exactly what he had been doing.

When we got home, he told the boys to go upstairs and me to go help my mom set the table. I hung back a little to see where my dad was going to put that bottle.

I watched him get it out of the car trunk and stash it in a corner of the garage. (A hoarder's dream, that garage... clutter upon clutter. My dad was very smart, and a even a bit of a scientist. He was always creating things, making things, collecting things. Anyway, he was a hoarder.)

That night after dinner, I watched him go downstairs and out to the garage.

I had heard my brothers talking about how their friends down the street would steal liquor and sell it to the older kids. This gave me the bright idea to steal my dad's bottle and sell it—that way he couldn't drink it. That's what I was gonna do.

The next morning before school I went down to the garage real early. I grabbed the bottle, put it in my book bag, and went down to the bus stop. One of my brothers' friends was there.

"Hey, I've got a bottle of vodka. Wanna buy it?" The guy was like, "Heck, yeah!" and I sold it to him for probably two dollars.

Later that night, the whole thing blew up. My dad got home from work, and not 15 minutes later he came into the kitchen, fucking LIVID. We didn't know why, and of course, he couldn't say. But I knew.

He pulled my brothers aside and asked down-low, "Who took my goddamn liquor?" My brothers had no idea, and of course, they would never think of me, being the sweet little kid sister. So my brothers got a whooping for it.

I stole another vodka bottle and sold it. I think I only did it twice, because I did not like what happened afterwards. My brothers were getting blame for it, and they kept accusing each other. I finally told them what I did, crying and saying I did it because I didn't want our dad to drink and I didn't know how to stop him.

Stuff like that was pushing me to the edge, even as a young kid. It had definitely pushed my mom to the edge. She wanted to leave my dad many, many times but could never bring herself to do it.

She decided to take us all on a train trip to go see her mom in Michigan, so she could think things through up there. So we all got on this train: my mom, me, and my three older hooligan brothers. I remember crawling up and down like monkeys all over the seats, just laughing and laughing with my brothers. Mom was ready to pull her hair out. She couldn't keep us all under control...she never could.

That summer was one of the coolest times I ever remember, a really great memory for me. Whenever there's a summer rain and I'm out in the middle of it, I get a memory of being in the front yard of my grandma's big house on the lawn, with the warm rain pouring down all over me, just dancing and singing in the rain. That was an amazing summer.

Then we went back home to the same old every-day, and my brothers started acting up again. Chris and Buff were always in trouble, or it sure seemed like they were. Smoking pot or maybe breaking and entering... and that meant more chaos at home. My mom was trying to deal with all of these boys who were always getting in trouble, plus a drunk husband. Pure chaos.

By then, my dad was well-known as Dick Gaines, The Neighborhood Drunk Dude. My mother was in a bit of a shell, constantly embarrassed by the things he'd do. The two of them would go out to dinner to their favorite pizza parlor and he would get rip-roaring drunk. Sometimes it was funny, because they had a big organ in the restaurant and my dad would get drunk and stupid and play it. At least he was a good singer. Mom was not quite so amused, but she never stood up to him.

Mom also left the job of disciplining the children to my dad. Some evenings, he would come home from work and sit in the living room, have a few beers, and try to relax. My brothers would come home after getting in some kind of trouble, and Mom would say to them, "Tell Dad what happened." None of them ever confessed to what they had done, so there was just silence. After a while, my dad would say, "Come into the bedroom because you're getting the belt." "The belt" was a thick brown leather belt with notches in it and a big buckle.

Over time, my brothers knew it was just best to lay still on the bed and take the beating. They had learned that fighting back just made it worse. And so I would hear my brothers screaming, and crying, and screaming, and it always scared me so bad.

It wasn't really talked about that much. I would hear those sounds and get scared, and then the next day would come and I would go to school, and *whatever,* just not think about it. I was just the tall, thin girl who everyone thought was "happy."

People knew about our family, and they sure liked to gossip about it. There was always talk on the neighborhood street like, "Oh, there's Dick Gaines. I wonder if he's drunk." Or, "Oh, Dick Gaines, he's the town drunk." That made me feel really bad.

What was weird was that my dad also had a reputation for being really creative at things. He was a very talented builder. One day we came home from school and my dad said he had a surprise for us. He had built these stilts and showed us how to use them. The next thing you know, there's a bunch of kids walking up and down the street on stilts my dad had built.

One windy day, we wanted to fly kites but couldn't afford to buy any. So my dad said, "Well, why don't we make some kites right now? I've got some little skinny stakes here. Go to your mom's room and get some wrapping paper." We were all wondering, *How do you make a kite out of wrapping paper?*

So we watched him get out his glue and these little teeny things that were almost like chopsticks. He glued them together, then glued the wrapping paper onto the stakes, and attached a kite string made out of sewing thread. I thought it was genius. Those were the great qualities of my dad. He made us laugh.

Another time I remember coming home one night and there were a bunch of men around our kitchen table, which was covered with clear jars of hot peppers and pickled onions. There were a lot of beer bottles on the table, and the guys were all red-faced, with sweat on their brows.

"Dad, what are you doing?" I couldn't figure out what was going on. That's when

I learned what a pepper-eating contest was. The men would go around the table, take a pepper out of the jar, eat it, and keep going around until someone couldn't do it anymore. That man would be eliminated. They'd keep going until there was only one pepper-eater left. Just another random thing that happened in my house. Flash to real-time... one of my brothers is now a hot-pepper connoisseur who makes the hottest chili powder, heat-infused jams, and salsas to blow your socks off!

My family, we all loved each other; there just wasn't a whole lot of direction or guidance for the kids and we all kinda got lost because of it. My parents did the best they could, but they just didn't know how to do it. There were bad times, but there were plenty of good times, too.

· 4 ·

The Great Cough Medicine Caper

Remember the story back at the beginning about the horrible Mr. Burlein, my fifth-grade teacher who I said would go to hell? There were some other things about the fifth grade that happened, and some of those things probably set me on a very bad path for the future.

In the early '70s, me and the neighborhood kids would sometimes walk to school. Most of the time we caught the bus. While we waited, we'd play Peewee football with little teeny plastic footballs, or maybe baseball, whichever sport was in season. There were also recreation programs after school, so we'd stay after and play foosball or kickball until it was time to go home. I loved being active, and that was a big positive for me.

One of the big negatives was my brothers smoking pot. I found their stash one day, which I thought was just yellow cigarettes. (I found out later it was pot wrapped in lemon papers.) I took one and put it in my book bag, and went to find my friend Barb, who was something of a "bad girl." I ran up to her and looked around to make sure no one saw us.

"Hey! Come on, let's go behind the bathrooms and smoke this," I whispered, like it was some big secret mission or something. I didn't even really know what it was, but I was pretty sure it was a joint. *Oh, my God, drugs in the fifth grade?*

We found some matches and lit the joint. First off, we hated the smell. We each took a puff, and we hated it so we put it out and threw it away. I guess I was trying to be like my older brothers, who were just out of control then. Not the greatest role models, but they were what they were.

Around that time, I was 11. My dad's drinking was increasing, and my mom's tolerance for it was decreasing. My mom was getting more angry and was just worn out from his alcoholism. I think she tried to leave him again, but he was so charming and she believed he wanted to stop. He always talked her into coming back.

Being a little older and understanding things a little better, I started wondering why he drank so much. There must have been *something* good about it because he did it so much. On the other hand, I could see the damage it was doing to my mom and that was definitely not good. I remember thinking, *How can I stop my dad from drinking?* Well, I had tried stealing and selling it, and that didn't work. Maybe I could try and get all the alcohol out of the house without him knowing? I knew where the liquor cabinet was.

So my Great Plan was to start by emptying out the cough medicine bottles and fill them with dad's Crème de Menthe. Then I planned to take the "cough medicine" to school to get it away from the house. I sure didn't want to get caught with liquor at school, so I drank it. And that's when it started, in fifth grade.

· 5 ·

WHAT THE BABYSITTER KNEW

When you start getting into your teenage years, you always need money for this and that, so I started babysitting around the neighborhood. My most regular customers were the people down the street. They had a pretty-but-older house with a pool, and two kids to babysit. The wife was nice enough, but the husband was a little bit *off*. I'll call him Calvin.

Around this time we started getting strange phone calls at home. I remember one time I answered the phone and I heard this man's voice say—real hushed—"Do you know who this is?" and then he started breathing hard. You know, back then "breathing hard" was like an obscene phone call.

So I said, "Who is this?" and he would hang up and call again the next day. I started getting creeped out because I was babysitting all alone. *Maybe this creepy-caller guy was following me around.*

Meanwhile, Calvin was being his weird self. I was babysitting his kids one day and he showed up at home when he was supposed to be at work. Another time, he was asking me what I did during school lunchtime and asked me to "come over and play, or we can talk." *Yeah, right.* I was still pretty naïve then.

So I was still getting these obscene phone calls at home. I finally told Mom, and she said that next time it happened we were going to call the police. Well, it happened again and Mom got on the other phone and demanded to know who was calling. He hung up. Mom called the police and they tapped our phone. They figured out it was *Calvin*, the weird guy whose kids I was babysitting. He was arrested. His wife was so mortified that she divorced him. Funny how I didn't remember that incident until just recently.

There were many adventures in my babysitting career. I used to watch our mailman's twins. I can remember holding his babies and I don't think I ever was able to tell them apart. My friend would come over and we'd snoop through the house and play hide-and-seek while the babies were sleeping. We'd poke around for good places to hide. The next thing you know my friend was like, "Oh my God, Heather, come here, come up here!" I went upstairs and see that she had found a secret panel in their upstairs room which had all of these grow lights and like 20 pot plants in there! *The mailman?!*

We bravely decided to pick some of the pot leaves and microwave them to see if we could get stoned. She liked smoking pot, but I wasn't sure if I liked it yet.

In seventh grade, I was still regularly bringing the Crème de Menthe "cough medicine" to school in my lunchbox, or book bag, or whatever. When I first started back in fifth grade, I sipped it, and it took a long time to empty out the bottles. But by seventh grade, I would go into the girl's restroom and just chug it. Oh, my God, that was amazing!! I loved the feeling after the first chug. And I knew nobody could smell it on me because it just smelled like mint. That was when the serious sneaking really started, and by then it was much more about getting liquor for myself rather than getting it away from my dad.

In spite of all that sneaky behavior, I was still pretty innocent. I was in love (!) with Sonny Valeri. He used to dress like a grown businessman and was a very nice boy. He asked if he could call me. Of course, then we had the phone on the wall with the big long cord (that was long before cell phones). He asked me to be his girlfriend and I was more than OK with that. I remember talking to him forever on the phone. We probably were boyfriend/girlfriend for maybe a week, and then it was like done. You know, seventh-grade innocent love... but Sonny really stuck with me. One of the good guys.

· 6 ·

COLD DUCK

By the eighth grade, I was officially a teenager. Somewhere I had gotten the notion that becoming a teenager was my license to start officially partying.

Two of my girlfriends told me about a dance that was coming up one Saturday in the fall, and they thought it would be fun to get some beers or some alcohol for before the dance. Well, that was the best idea ever!

My oldest brother, Buff, and his girlfriend were up from San Diego for a visit. The day of the dance, she styled my hair for me (actually, she teased the shit out of it). She also let me borrow her trendy "Candies" platform shoes. Who could forget Candies? I was so excited!

Anyway, I had asked my brother to get us a pint of liquor before the dance. He at first said no way, but I begged and begged until he finally caved, on one condition: I had to promise—all us girls had to promise—that if we got caught, we would not ever tell who got it for us. We had to say we found it somewhere, like in a bush or something. We could not tell!!

Buff said, "If you say I got it, it will be over your dead bodies," and we were like, "Cross our hearts! Hope to die!" I think we would have given him a kidney if he had asked for it.

He gave us a ride to the dance and on the way, we stopped at the liquor store. Forbidden thrills! Then we saw Buff come out of the liquor store with three bottles of Cold Duck. *Cold Duck, WTF!* If you don't know what Cold Duck is, it's a mix of cheap red wine and domestic sparkling wine, probably two dollars a bottle. Awful stuff.

So my friends and I were sitting in the back seat, drinking our Cold Duck right out of the bottle. Well, me being the "fruit doesn't fall far from the alcoholic tree," I chugged mine to the bottom, like lickety-split. My friends still had half a bottle left. They were asking me to help them finish theirs... I don't even know how much I had in all, but it was a lot. I loved the taste of it.

We brushed our teeth and started chewing gum to cover the winey smell. I teetered and tottered on my Candies up to the school, and into the dark gym. (Trust me, someone who isn't used to wearing heels shouldn't be teetering on them, let alone be drunk-teetering.) The lights were dancing on the ceiling, with all the girls on one side, all the boys on the other.

All of a sudden the gym started spinning, and then I said something like, "Oh my God, I think I'm going to PUKE!" So I went for the trash can. I threw up again and again, and somehow found my way to the girl's room to wash up. I teetered back out, trying to play it cool. *Nothing to see here, folks!*

I tottered past the teacher who supervised the Recreation Club I was in, and he asked me how I was feeling.

"GREAT! Ower*you*?" I slurred. He asked me if I'd been drinking and I slurred some more, "No, shir." He asked me again if I was OK, and at that point I was still sober enough to figure out that he was onto me. "Gotta go, sheeya later!" I said, and stumbled off.

I made it back over to my friends and frantically told them that we had to get out of there. Somehow my brother came to pick us up, wondering how we could be so shitfaced and still be standing.

We got home, I got in bed and immediately started throwing up again, sending Cold Duck-vomit all over the sheets, the bedspread, everywhere. My parents were still asleep, and thankfully they stayed that way while my brothers got me in the shower and put the sheets in the washer. They had my back. I just hoped my parents wouldn't find out.

Sunday, I caught up with my Cold-Duck girlfriends and they were both feeling *so* bad. I was, too. That was my first experience with a hangover. We all said we were never, ever, ever going to drink again! We all swore, cross our heart. *Ha!* Famous not-so-last words.

It was back to school on Monday and everything was cool until the principal called me into the office. Good ol' Mr. Bentley. Nice on the outside, out-to-get-you on the inside.

"Is there anything you'd like to tell me about the dance on Saturday night?" he asked.

Of course, I said, "No, sir," because everybody knew me to be this innocent, sweet nice girl. I was even a cheerleader in the eighth grade. (To this day I have no idea how I made the cheerleading squad because I didn't have the coordination or the coolness.)

"You went to the dance?" He was going to persist with this. I had to acknowledge that I was there, and he stared me down and said, "I heard you were drinking."

I said as innocently as I could, "NO, not me. What are you talking about?" When you're young you think you can get away with stuff like that.

"Heather, tell me the truth. You're not going to get in trouble, I just need to know." He was always nice to me, so I said I had a little bit to drink. Big mistake.

"Heather I should kick you off the cheerleading team." *Oh no, no!* I would never live that down. I begged him, "Please, please don't, please don't do that!"

He must have felt sorry for me so he backed off and said I wouldn't be kicked off the team—but that some kind of disciplinary action had to be taken. He didn't tell me what that would be.

On Tuesday, I came home from class and was having an after-school snack when my mom walked in, carrying the mail. She opened one of the letters and started reading it. I was watching her reading, watching her face go straight, pure white, like somebody had died.

"Shit, shit shit!!!" she yelled. I had NEVER heard my mom cuss, not ever. She threw the letter down and ran out of the room. Somebody had to have died.

I slowly walked over to pick up the letter, which started off:

Dear Mrs. Gaines,

We regret to inform you that your daughter, Heather, was intoxicated at the school dance on Saturday night

blah blah blah

Everything after that was meaningless. I WANTED TO DIE!! I never, ever wanted to hurt my mom; she didn't deserve that terror from me. The last thing she needed was another drunk or another troublemaker kid in the family.

I summoned all my courage to go find her. I hated it when she cried; it hurt my heart. I found her in her bedroom. She was crying.

"Heather, I'm so disappointed in you. How could you do this? When did you start drinking? I am so upset with you!" She was crying while she was trying to talk. It was terrible.

I just kept saying, "I'm sorry, Mom, I'm sorry, Mom, I'll never do it again!" I must have said it 10 times. When I think about that now, I can only wonder how much I must have sounded like my dad, saying I wasn't going to drink anymore.

She finally started to calm down, and I asked her if she was going to tell my dad. "No, I am not," she said. I was so relieved. I couldn't stand the thought of letting my dad down, too. Not to mention that I was scared of getting in trouble.

"I'm not going to tell him," she repeated. "*You* are. As soon as he comes home." I was hysterical, pleading with her not to make me do that. She said, "You've made your bed now you will lie in it!" *Holy shit, I'm gonna get The Belt, like my brothers always did.* I thought about running away in that instant.

She looked me right in the eyes and I knew that now she was getting to the nitty gritty. "Tell me where you got it, Heather," she demanded. Remembering that I had crossed my heart and hoped to die if I found myself in this situation, I told her, "I found it in a bush."

After about 20 minutes of "You did not!" and "Yes, I did!" she started getting really pissed off. "GODDAMMIT, Heather, you had better tell me right this minute!" Her cussing again meant she was really serious.

"OK... OK, we got it at the liquor store." I had to confess. Then she asked who bought it, and we went back and forth for a while between "Who bought it?" and "I don't know!" I had sworn not to tell on Buff. I could not tell on Buff.

She said, "I know you're lying and you're going to be restricted for a year if you don't tell me the truth. Tell me right now, Heather!" I was 14. I couldn't be restricted for a year; that was unheard of. It was like a death sentence for an eighth-grader.

Buff had gone back to San Diego the day after the dance, so for a second I thought I could get away with saying it was him because he was so far away. I had *sworn* I wouldn't tell, but I couldn't think of a good lie, either. I went back and forth in my head a dozen times. *How can I get out of this??*

I finally confessed that Buff had bought it for us. She was livid, yelling about how she was going to have him arrested for contributing to the delinquency of a minor. I didn't even know what that meant.

Mom called him up and she started shouting at him. "I am calling the police and having you arrested!" I was pulling on the phone, screaming, "No, mom, no mom!!" She hung up on him. I knew for sure that my own brother was going to kill me.

My dad came home that night and Mom told him all of what had happened. To my surprise, he talked her out of pressing any charges, but Buff did not come back up to visit for a long time.

There was still this business that I had to tell my dad that I got drunk at the dance. I was terrified to tell him, but there must have been some real remorse in my voice because he took it a lot better than I thought he was going to. He wasn't happy or OK with it, don't get me wrong. The look on his face was sheer disappointment—and fright. He was scared and he was sad.

He pleaded with me, "Heather, please don't do this. Please do not drink again."

"But Daddy, you drink," I said.

He replied, "Yes, but I'm old enough. You are not."

I apologized to him three or four times. I never wanted to disappoint my dad, ever.

· 7 ·

BY POPULAR DEMAND

As you know, in the '70s all the California girls had long, straight hair. I had this crazy mess of curly hair. I never felt cute. Everybody always looked at my cute friends; nobody looked at me, nobody asked me out. I always felt kind of left out a little bit going into the school dance. No one would ask me to dance.

I thought maybe trying out for cheerleading again might get some of the football guys to like me, so I decided to try out for the junior varsity squad. I guess I was pretty good because I was the first girl in school history to make the varsity team as a ninth-grader.

So there was something I was good at, I guess. I was stoked, like, *Oh, my God, I have arrived. I'm going to finally be popular!*

In ninth grade, there were breaks between classes, then lunch and two more classes, and we were done. So I started smoking pot on school breaks, then I would smoke pot before school and go to class. My second class was typing, the best grade I ever got. That cracks me up.

After typing class, I'd go to "The Hill," where everybody went and smoked pot and cigarettes. I became one of the "Hill People." At lunch break, we would meet back at The Hill, have some Chablis and smoke some more pot. It was my way of trying to fit in and be accepted. (It would not be until much, much later on that I would realize the danger of all that early exposure to drugs and alcohol.)

Aside from the home situation, I thought life was pretty good. I had friends, I was swimming, I was cheerleading, and I liked the California life. There was even a couple of small earthquakes that year, but nothing like what was about to crack my whole life wide open.

· 8 ·

The Call

My Aunt Bonnie would fly out to California and visit us a couple of times a year. She was from Virginia Beach, and she and my mom were pretty tight. They would stay up late and talk in the kitchen, probably about how unhappy my mom was.

Not too much by accident, Mom said I could go back to Virginia Beach with Aunt Bonnie and stay for a couple of weeks. That would be cool because I really liked my aunt and especially my cousin Carolyn. The problem was that I had cheerleading practice. My mom assured me that I would get back in time, and she thought it would be good for me to get away and hang out with my cousin for a while. Really, I think she wanted some space of her own for a little bit. So I went.

My cousin Carolyn swam on the local country club team and asked me to swim with her. That was kind of cool because I was still doing swimming even though I was busy with cheerleading. I was fast and beat everybody on that swim team.

They all wanted me to join up, but it was a country club, and you had to be a member. I was definitely not the country-club type. People around there wore funny clothes. They were all preppy alligators on polo shirts, pink and green, seersucker, debutantes, cotillions... all these things this small-town girl had never heard of. I was different and didn't fit into this scenario, not at all.

Two days before I was supposed to leave Aunt Bonnie's and Virginia Beach behind, my mom called.

"Heather, I need to talk to you," she said, in a way that started to make my stomach hurt.

She said, "I finally decided to leave your dad."

What? WHAT? I was especially shocked because like I said before, I had always been my mom's sounding board, so you'd figure I'd know about this. Turns out her BFF, Winnie, helped her make that decision without my input.

She told me, "I'm giving you kids the choice: You can either decide to live with me, or live with your dad." Complete, huge silence. *What do you mean live with you or Dad??*

My mom explained that she was moving to Virginia with my little sister Elizabeth and was going to stay with her sister Bonnie. The boys were going to stay with Dad.

"So, what do you want to do, Heather?" She already knew the answer; she knew I wouldn't go live with my dad because his drinking was getting worse and worse. My relationship with him was getting more difficult, and that hurt me. My dad was still the apple of my eye; I just couldn't live with him.

It was like a game show and I had 30 seconds to decide... tick tock tick tock...

I just blurted out, "Of course, I'll live with you!! But I have to come home first and get my stuff." She told me I couldn't come home, which sent me into a hysterical crying rant. "What do you mean? What about all my swimming trophies? My posters? What about my best friends? What about my cheerleading?" I was fighting back so many tears. It was way too much to handle all at once.

Then she said she and Elizabeth were leaving the day after tomorrow, so I had to decide right then. *WTF!!!* I thought my life was over. I mean *over*. I was in ninth grade. Your friends and your stuff and your life is everything at that age.

"Hold on, I'll put your dad on," she said. This was more than I could take. Now I was in shock, everything was happening so fast. Aunt Bonnie was standing there watching me cry, not knowing what to do.

So my dad got on the phone. "Hey, Hooch. I love you very much."

All I could say was, "This is a nightmare. This can't be real. I love you Dad, I love you Dad ..." I was just crying and crying and crying. I didn't even know if I would ever see my dad again.

Just like that, POOF, my family was broken. I was pissed off at my mom, I was so damn sad about the whole thing and pretty much in total despair. That event left a huge mark and set the tone for the crazy rest of my life.

For a while, I just sat there thinking about my dad, and how much I loved him but how much I didn't want to live with him because his drinking had gotten so bad. It was a terribly confusing time in my life.

· 9 ·

A Round Peg in a Square Hole

Moving to Virginia was a huge culture shock. I was a 15-year-old who was thrust into a life she didn't know, with cousins she didn't really remember. Out of nowhere it was private schools and a country-club atmosphere. Nobody in Virginia smoked pot or drank, I was sure of that. Before I left California, I was smoking pot every day! I was going to be an alien on a distant planet, a puzzle piece that didn't belong. Worse than that, even.

Just when I thought I was starting to be somebody in California, now we were moving to this new town and a new school all the way across the country. I had been all ready to be one of the popular girls because I was the first ninth-grader to go into the 10th grade as a varsity cheerleader. I thought for sure I would be one of the popular kids. I might get a boyfriend, I might get a date. Having to move was a kick in the stomach. I *hated* it.

One of the worst things was not having all of my worldly possessions, the things I had to leave in California: all my trophies, my Mark Spitz and David Partridge posters. I was just kind of left empty. Fifteen years old, no friends, new school, no nothing. *Ugh.*

So now we were in Virginia Beach, in this house I thought was a mansion: a huge two-story colonial house with big white columns. Four bedrooms, three bathrooms. I was living with my aunt, uncle, and three cousins; my mom had left my dad after 25 years of marriage and was bringing her best friend and my little sister. It was a very full house.

Poor Elizabeth. She was in the middle of everything, not knowing what the fuck was going on, being pulled here and pulled there and pulled here and pulled there. I had empathy for her, you know. It was tough because I was trying to find my own way, so I understood how it felt. My mom was doing the best that she could, but I'll never forget the look of bewilderment on my little sister's face during that time.

If you remember, I was a swimmer from a very young age, so at least I could swim at the country club with my younger cousins. I pretty much just latched on to their life, but it was so different! They dressed different. You know, I'd never heard of Oshkosh B'gosh pants. They were cool corduroys. And they always wore a cardigan-like pullover cable-knit sweaters and they had alligators and polo ponies on their shirts. Button-down Oxfords. I hadn't worn *any* of that. I just wore hip-hugger bell bottoms and had my hair long and curly and crazy.

Going into the 10th grade was lonely and kind of scary. My cousins went to the private school that was next to my high school. East Armistead High School, Home of the Patriots. I came from Home of the Bulldogs! Who makes a boring person their mascot? Yep, hated it!

There was one good thing: I discovered that one of my cousins liked to drink, so we would sneak around together sometimes. It was like my old California days! We would take beers out of the fridge and hide them in the doghouse for the weekend. Sometimes we would crawl out our bedroom window, down onto the lower roof, and jump down and sneak out.

We stayed with Aunt Bonnie for a while, then we finally found a place for the winter after Mom found a job. It was just a few houses off the beach. I was really excited about that because now I could be the beach girl I'd always wanted to be in California; I could go down to the beach whenever I wanted. That was one of the few pluses in my brain, besides sneaking drinks with my cousin.

Mom was struggling as a single parent, just trying to do the best she could. She worked for Social Services and took the bus to work. I think she didn't like it, because, you know, that was kind of demeaning for her. But the one really good thing about my mom leaving my dad after 25 years was to get herself back. She took a lot of emotional abuse for a lot of years, but when she got away from it, I could sit back and watch her get younger and younger. She got more hip with her clothes. She changed her hairstyle. Next thing you know, she was finding things she was interested in. It was like this lady living in a black-and-white movie who finally broke through that screen and was in living Technicolor.

That was one of the best things about moving to Virginia, but I still missed my brothers. I felt sorry for them because they were with my dad in California. But we all had a choice. Later, Dink would say that was the hardest choice he'd ever had to make in his life.

· 1 O ·

Amy

One day at the bus stop, I was just standing there by myself and this girl came up to me and said, "Hi, my name's Amy." She was barely five feet tall.

"Hi, I'm Heather," I answered, checking her out. She said she hadn't seen me before, and I told her I had just moved there from California. I was kind of emphasizing the "moved here from California" part like it made me kind of cool or something, but I wasn't. I was scared. I was afraid of being in my own skin. I knew I wasn't going to fit in. I knew the school was going to be huge. I knew I wasn't going to be able to find my locker. I knew I wasn't going to find my classes. I was petrified.

I got on the bus, and I didn't know what to do. *Where to sit? Back, front... am I going to take someone's seat?* So Amy and I started talking. She told me she lived a block away. They had a house on the beach and she had a brother, too. We became fast friends.

Amy had her whole clique of her own. Her best friend at the time was Lila Seaberg, and the three of us became like The Musketeers. That triangle of friends made things a little less scary for me even though I still felt out of the loop of the world.

I really don't remember a whole lot about my classes in 10th grade. I wasn't a good student, just a C student because I could never concentrate on my schoolwork.

I did start meeting more people and stuff and it was all right, but I missed my dad a lot. He and I would talk about once a week. He would ask me how school was and things like that. And we kept a pretty good relationship until the time I went out to visit him, a surprise visit. After that, I think he and I only spoke on holidays, and that was because he broke my heart. More about that later.

In the 10th grade, it was time to start Driver's Ed! We had a really cool instructor who would teach you to drive, and then he didn't care where you went. I got to be a pretty good student, I guess. When it was my turn to drive, we would go down to the beach to my house and get the newspaper, and then we'd drive back to school. And that was cool.

I remember when it was time for me to turn 16 and both Amy and Lila were really happy. I would be the first one of us to get my license, and pretty soon we could all tool around in Amy's car. Amy's mom gave her this huge station wagon we called the "tuna boat" because it was so big. Amy had to sit on a pillow to see out the windshield.

Before the driving test, I studied, studied, and studied. Like I said, I was never good in school and choked on taking tests. I had bad comprehension because I had bad concentration. I was always daydreaming in school, wanting to be somewhere else. Wanting to be someone else. And drinking more and more to drown that feeling out.

Finally my mom took me for my final driving test, the one that determines whether or not you get your license. Guess what, I failed it! I failed a lot of things back then, but that was a big one.

That was on a Friday and the girls were all looking forward to me driving us all to parties and whatever that weekend. So of course, I went down a notch in the friend group. I finally got my license after the third try.

· 11 ·

The BFD About the DMV ID

Around that time, I heard people talking about having two licenses, one real, and one not. Didn't everyone have a fake ID in high school? You had to have one to go to the bars, right? I found out how to get one and I planned to use my older cousin's name. I screwed up my courage to go to the DMV with all of the information I needed to get my fake license, nervous as all hell, and who was there but my older cousin, whose name I was using to get the fake ID! *Fuck me.* I turned and ran so fast out of that DMV, and never did get the fake ID.

It was also normal to cut class, and so one day my friends and I decided to skip school. They said it was easy, just forge a note and put the secretary's name on it. They'd done it plenty of times, so I wasn't worried.

So we skipped school and went to the mall. We were on our way over to the McDonald's and who do we see but my *Aunt Bonnie.* Fuck, every time I tried to take a shortcut or break the rules, I always got caught. I always seem to get caught. I felt like the DORK of the group.

The next day I had to turn my "absence note" in, and now I was paranoid. I had my note, which was terrible, because I have the worst handwriting in the world. My circles, zeros, and exes were never right because I had to use my left hand. (I broke my right arm in kindergarten and my hand was in a cast forever.) Never did learn how to do it right.

"Who signed this?" said the office lady. She wasn't having it. I had signed it with the name of Cheryl Caudill. "This is not Cheryl's signature," she said, glaring right through me. *Busted.*

Usually, it wouldn't be the worst thing if I got caught, because if I got caught, then I would be suspended, and getting suspended meant I would have to stay home, which meant I could spend the day at the beach because my mom worked. So that would be all right, except that this incident happened to come right when they started doing "in-school suspension."

I learned that I was officially suspended, and that I would be one of the first people to do the new in-school detention. DAMN! I had my day all planned, just like Ferris Bueller. I was going to go to the beach, I was going to watch all my shows. I was going to do everything and just go back to bed.

But no. I was ordered to show up at a certain room at 7:30 a.m. *So, what do I bring?* I asked. *Bring lunch, they said.* So I walked into the detention room, and the first person I saw looked like a big, brown brick wall, like a retired NFL football player. He scared the living dog doo out of me. There were four other students there besides me.

He growled, "Now, you're all going to sit down, and you're going to do what I say." He gave us busy-work to do, and then it was time for lunch. *Great, so I'll take my lunch and go sit with my friends.*

Then Mr. NFL Player said, "When we go to lunch, we're going to walk in a straight line and there will be a table for all of us. We're all sitting together." Oh, my God, how humiliating for all of my friends to see me sitting at The Dork Table.

So I got through that school suspension, and I never got suspended again. I never even cut school again, except when I knew I was really going to get away with it, like Senior Skip Day.

You'd think from all this delinquent behavior that I was raised in a barn, but I was brought up with *some* values. We sat down for dinner every night, and we always said *Yes, ma'am, no, ma'am.* My family always hugged each other, said "I love you" all the time, and kissed each other goodbye. It was the strangest combination of love and trouble and chaos.

· 12 ·

On the "Up" Escalator

When the public-school kids were getting ready to go to the junior prom, my cousins were getting ready for Cotillion. If you've never heard of that, it's a fancy ball where the girls (debutantes) are "presented to society." My oldest cousins were becoming debutantes, and I got invited to all the parties. But it was almost like "always the bridesmaid, never the bride." I didn't have a boyfriend to go to these parties with.

I haven't mentioned anything about high-school dating, and there's a reason for that. I never had a date in high school. My high-school friends who are reading this book probably don't believe that. But believe it. I never had a date in high school. I was just kind of like everybody's "friend."

I was constantly sad and depressed. You know, hiding it, though. I felt like the cool girls were all very pretty and I was just kind of like the dull one, hidden in the woodwork. I was a tall girl, what they used to call a carpenter's dream: flat as a board, skinny as a nail! Everybody else was "developing" except for me. I was just growing taller. And of course, you know, my legs were so long that nothing fit right. I was always trying to be cute but never succeeding, because I was kind of like a mix of preppy and beachy, which was just weird. That made me feel like an outcast and an oddball.

That is when I learned to fake it so I could try and measure up with the "in" crowd. They would invite me to different functions and stuff, but I never felt like I truly ever belonged. I really didn't. I felt like any day they were going to drop me because I just didn't have any confidence.

I remember this one party I got invited to. Amy was seeing this guy named Dan Wrentham. He was cool, and really, really funny. They let me tag along as a third wheel.

Dan had a gold-ish Charger, not even gold, actually—I think it was puke-orange because we used to say "the puke orange car that Dan drives." We went to a party at this rich kid's house, funny because his name was Rich. He was one of the hottest guys in school, and I always had a crush on him. (You'll hear more about that name later on.)

By this time, I was drinking vodka more than ever. No one could believe how much I could drink and not really get drunk. I thought it was pretty cool to be able to drink everyone under the table and not throw up... it must have been in my genes.

It was time to leave the party, and we all piled in the car, and I started thinking, *Oh my God, I feel kinda sick.* Amy and Dan were in the front and sure enough, I started throwing up in the back. Dan was yelling, "Not in my car! Not in my car!" I threw up all over the floor of his backseat. To this day, I think he still remembers that.

That year, me and Amy and Lila were supposed to be in this parade, and we were gonna be clowns. Amy and Lila got ready together, but they left me out. (I think there was a little jealousy there... Lila didn't like me "stealing" her best friend.) The two of them had their cool-ass matching clown costumes and I didn't know how to make mine. I ended up getting a hula hoop and putting a sheet over it. I painted myself as a sad clown and we walked through the parade.

I remember seeing a picture of that parade in the yearbook, and how I felt so alone in the midst of so many people. The face of that clown was truly how I felt in my heart. I was sad. I missed my California friends and for me, Virginia was really hard.

But my senior year was coming, and there was a lot more crazy stuff to come. The funny thing was, when I got to be a senior, I started feeling a little better about myself and started getting invited to more parties. I was pretty funny then, with a sarcastic sense of humor.

When it came time for the yearbook nominations for Best Dressed and Most Likely To Succeed, well, that was not me. I actually did get nominated for Class Clown and all my people were going, Oh, you're going to win that! I really didn't understand why. I mean, I knew I was funny, but I didn't think anybody paid any attention to me. In the end, I didn't win it. But it was kind of cool to be nominated.

That year, I started drinking quite a bit at parties. I used to keep beers or liquor in my closet. My mom would find my stash, and she would be like, "Oh, my God, Heather." I could hear the disappointment. Fear, too, because she didn't want me to end up like my dad.

Mom blamed Amy for corrupting me, which we still laugh about today. (We all know who corrupted who.) We're still best friends, you know, but there was a time—a long time—when Amy and I didn't talk. That was when she had to pull herself away from me because she saw me "killing myself" (her words) and she couldn't bear it.

The last year of high school was pretty much all fun/all the time. My brothers came to visit and I ended up going with them on the return trip to California. We called it the Double E Express, which stood for weed and speed. We did Virginia Beach to California in three days without stopping. I don't suggest that for anyone!! I even saw a UFO!

Three adults and my little niece in a Toyota pickup truck, what could go wrong? In the middle of that trip—in Cottonwood County, Tennessee, to be exact—I was driving along at three o'clock in the morning. My brothers were passed out, crashed from all the speed they were taking. It was definitely "good ol' boys" country, which I found out for sure when a state trooper pulled me over for speeding.

Now, the usual option when you're pulled over is something along the lines of, "Ma'am, I'm giving you a ticket and you can pay it at the courthouse... blah blah blah," Not with this guy! This guy was super-shady, and literally told me, "Follow me down this road, give ME $250 or you go to jail." No discussion, no good option. It was all of the money I had for my trip. FUCK!! I paid the cop and when we got to La Jolla, I don't think I talked to my brothers for a whole day.

I ended up staying in California for a little while. I met a blue-eyed, blonde surfer boy on the beach in La Jolla, but that's another story. At some point my mom called me and said I had to get back to school by the day after tomorrow or else I wasn't going to graduate. I had missed too many days of school already.

And so I had to go back. The cop had taken all of my money, but my brother's

LAST CALL IN CALI

You might be wondering about my dad. He was still in California, living in the house I grew up in, while we were in VB starting our awful new life. I decided during 10th grade that I wanted to go back and visit him, so I saved up my babysitting money and, with my Mom's approval, surprised my father with a visit.

You read that right. I arranged to have my friend Sandy pick me up at the airport and I hopped a plane on a Friday without telling my dad I was coming. Sounds like an adventure, right? I'm gonna surprise Dad! Fun! It was a surprise, all right.

Sandy picked me up as planned, and because her house was just four doors away from Dad's, I walked up the street to my old house and knocked on the door. I was so excited!

This guy answered the door—I had no idea who he was, but he looked pretty scary. Fat and sweaty with gray hair and a t-shirt that looked like it had food stains all over it. Ugh, it was disgusting. He sneered at me and asked, "Who are you?"

"Who the hell are you?" I snapped. "And where's my dad? I'm Heather." The dude let me in, and I was just shocked at what I saw.

Food and dirty dishes were piled up, ashtrays and cigarette butts were everywhere, and the entire house was messy and smelly. I was on the verge of tears. This can't be my house. What is going on here?

I finally ound my father, asleep in his bedroom. I woke him up pretty rudely.

"Oh my God, Heather, what are you doing here?" he said, barely comprehending what was going on. I was crying. "I saved up all my money to come and see you!", I said. I asked him who the gross scary dude was (it was his friend, Marty), and told him that he couldn't be there. I wanted to visit my Dad, not Marty.

He laughed and said, "It's fine, Heather, go to sleep and I'll see you in the morning."

Great. So I went into my old bedroom, and found another disaster. Could this get any worse? There was crap piled up everywhere. No sign of my favorite posters, my trophies, or my ribbons, until I spotted them stuffed away in the closet. It was all so dirty and disgusting and I was not staying there. (There was also the Gross Scary Dude to consider.)

So I climbed out of my bedroom window and walked back down the street to Sandy's house, hoping I could spend the night there. Sandy's mom let me in and was so nice to me. I was sobbing and I told her I had nowhere to go, and she let me stay.

The next morning, I called Dad and told him Gross Scary Dude had to go and that the house had to be cleaned before I would come over. Pretty demanding for a high-school kid!

So Dad sent Marty on his way and cleaned up the place a bit. We hung out all day, went for a drive, and visited one of his friends. Nothing special, really. Then we went back to the house and drank some beer together. (I thought that was cool at the time, but wow, what responsible dad does that?). I went to bed feeling happy.

The next day, we hung out again pretty much like the day before. We had a great time, and got back to the house about three o'clock in the afternoon. Then Dad said he had to run an errand, but that he'd be back in a little bit.

"A little bit" turned out to be two days.

We talked on the phone two or three times during the time he was gone, doing who knows what. He kept saying he'd come back, but then he'd call and say, "Heather, I'm sorry, I just fell asleep. I'll be back in a while."

I kept waiting around for him to come back but he didn't show up 'til about ten o'clock on the last night I was there.

I was heartbroken. I only had a few days with my dad and he left me by myself in a dirty, broken-down house that was a shithole compared to the nice little home I knew as a kid. It was like he didn't even want to be around me. *Didn't I matter to him? Who does that to their own flesh-and-blood child?* It made me so angry, so upset, the way he treated me.

He finally came back, flinging a bunch of lies and excuses about where he'd been. I knew he'd been out drinking and was passed out somewhere, with little (make that no) thought to the well-being of his daughter. Of course, he was totally apologetic and kept telling me he loved me, but I was too upset at that point, so I left and went back down to Sandy's house. I seemed more welcome there than I was at my own childhood home.

I'm pretty sure I called my mom, crying, and she told me to just come home the next day. I was just devastated when I returned to Virginia Beach. From then on, when my father called, Mom would make me get on and talk with him—but I always cut it short.

"Hi Dad, love you, Dad…" and then I'd hand off the phone to someone else.

Over the next number of years, I talked to him on the phone but never saw him again in person. I was no longer daddy's girl, and he was no longer the apple of my eye.

Later on, years after his death, I would myself turn into that person with the dirty, messy house, that person with all the broken promises, the lost days and empty dreams. His treatment of me also had a serious effect on my relationships, as you will see.

girlfriend was nice enough to give me the plane fare home. My stomach was turning the whole way because I just didn't know what was coming next.

· 13 ·

PROM

Now it was time for Senior Prom.

I was lifeguarding at the Princeton Country Club. Most of my guy friends were there because they were my fellow workers. There was this guy named Joe Harman, and he and I became really good friends. He went to a private school, so I usually just saw him at work.

I thought one day, *Joe's fun to hang out with. Maybe I'll invite him to the prom.* So I gathered up all the courage I could and asked him if he would go to the prom with me.

"Yes, of course, I'll go with you," he said. *I was so happy.* I couldn't believe it. We weren't boyfriend/girlfriend or anything, just great friends. That was so awesome.

I immediately called Amy to tell her I had a date for the prom. She was stoked and said that Joe and I could go with her and her boyfriend. We were both so excited.

Well, a few days before the prom, Joe called me.

"Heather, I'm so sorry but I can't go to the prom." *What? I could not have heard that right.*

"Why not?" I asked, feeling kind of pissed off and hurt at the same time. He explained that he had to go out of town for a lacrosse tournament he "forgot about." He apologized again. (I still don't know if he really had a lacrosse game. My lack of ego and self-esteem said he probably just didn't want to go at the last minute and didn't know what to say to get out of it.)

So I was like, "Wow, all right, well, thanks for calling." *Thanks for calling to tell me you're dumping me as your prom date?*

I called Amy up and gave her the news. She promised she would find me another date.

There was a friend of a friend I used to surf with, and he had a brother who didn't have a prom date yet. I kind of knew this brother; his name was Louie. He wasn't in my circle and he wasn't really anybody that I would hang out with. He was just *meh*. So that was like the option of options of options.

I told my mom I needed to get a prom dress. Mom sewed a lot, so she said she would make me one. Back then there were sewing shops that had Butterick patterns. We headed off to the sewing shop and found the most amazing dress pattern. Of course, it was a Bob Mackie design. If you don't know who Bob Mackie was, he designed Cher's clothes. Very flashy. If my mom was alive today, she would call it "Heather's frontless/backless dress that was low in the front and low in the back and too low on both sides for a high-school senior."

We found some material, a kind of silver-bluish color. Mom made the dress and it was amazing. In the meantime, this guy Louie called me and asked, "Hey, do you want to go to prom?" (like this wasn't a big setup anyway) and I was like, "Sure, I'll go to prom with you."

"Well, what color's your dress?" he asked. I told him it was silver-blue and to make sure he got a silver-bluish tux, so we would match. That was the thing, you had to match.

The first time I met Louie was when he picked me up for prom. He just wasn't my type, but I was determined to go to prom because it was like, you *have* to go the prom, right?

So he picked me up, reeking of pot. I could tell he was very nervous even though he was stoned as hell. He showed up in a powder-blue tux, after asking me what color my dress was so we would match. "It's supposed to be silver-blue," I grumbled. I was picking at everything because I just didn't want to be with this guy.

We went and picked up Amy and her date to go to dinner first, which was going to be at the Ocean Point restaurant, where Amy's mom worked. We were all excited for a nice meal and one of the nicer restaurants on the water.

As we were pulling into the parking lot, Louie said, "Hey, let's smoke a joint!" Amy, her date, and I looked at each other and I guess he figured we didn't want to. And so Louie said, "Well, I'll meet you guys in there then. I'm just going to do a quick toke." I was like, *Oh, my fucking God, this is my life.*

PART II
YOUNG ADULTHOOD

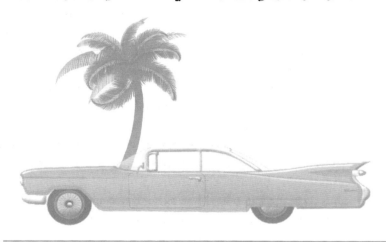

College (or not)

I graduated high school! Thank God!

During my senior year in 1979, everybody was thinking about what college they were going to, and this and that. I knew my grades probably weren't going to get me into anywhere. My SAT scores were very, very low because I think I got drunk the night before.

My mom said to try St. Augustine, try Appalachian State. Try Radford. So I applied to those colleges, and of course, I didn't get into any of them. My mom resigned herself to the fact that I was gonna be going to the local community college.

Lila had got into the University of Florida. So did some of my new friends, Melanie and Janine, who I met through a fellow lifeguard at the country club. (All the lifeguards were surfers, so I started hanging out with the surfer guys and girls.) Amy went off to Radford.

When I first started community college, I decided I was going to major in recreation. (It is a thing, you can do that.) I was thinking, Oh, I won't have to work too hard for a recreation degree. Then I thought better of it and decided that hotel restaurant management would be a smarter choice.

I think I had a job for a little bit—like a millisecond—as a waitress. Amy and I applied for jobs at the Magical Pancake House, a crazy, fast-paced breakfast diner on the strip. We both got hired, but I got fired pretty quick because I couldn't do the job. I wasn't fast enough and I couldn't understand the computerized cash register. Remember, me plus math equals ZERO! But in spite of everything, I killed at marrying the ketchups!

Everyone had gone off to school in Florida and I was at the community college in Virginia Beach, not knowing anyone. My classes were okay, I just wasn't into it at all. I remember being in the cafeteria and meeting up with these people who would bring beer to school, hang out in the cafeteria, drink their beers and play cards. Now I was like, I love love love college! I would go to a class, then go back to the cafeteria to drink beer and play cards.

Not a lot of schoolwork was getting done and my first semester grades were not great. My mom was telling me I had better shape up because she wasn't going to pay for me to just go and piss it away. I'm like, Okay, Mom. Okay, Mom. I so wanted to please her.

I was just playing around, drinking, having fun with people. That's when I met my awesome skateboarder friend, Elcee. I used to call him Elcee White, my black friend. It's probably not politically correct, but that's how it is. I really thought it was funny.

Elcee was skateboarding everywhere and wore Vans skater shoes. There were skater boys and surfers everywhere in those days. It was a blast. I met more new people, like Dustin, a friend of Elcee's. He had one of those little Toyota Love trucks with a camper on the back. I remember one night we all were gonna have a party, but we couldn't figure out how or where to get a keg.

The party was going to be at Elcee's house because his parents were out of town. Dustin said, "Hey, I'm a member of the F.O.P. (Fraternal Order of Police). "I know how to break in and get a keg." Are you serious?

I'm not going to say where we did this, but we hopped the fence, broke in and got a keg! Time to hightail it back to Elcee's! I couldn't believe we got away with it. Dustin said it was OK, all we had to do was return the keg. So the next night we had to break back in and return the empty keg. And we did. All just fun college stuff.

Mom paid for the next three semesters, I think. Not the best investment, because I ended up failing out of the fourth semester.

Around this time I was missing my friends who had gone off to school. Lila and Melanie would come home for the summers and rent the upstairs of a house Lila's dad owned, so we hung out there a lot. There was a bunch of surfer guys renting the downstairs apartment, and we partied with them whenever we could. That's where I met Russ, who you'll hear about later. We called it the "3700 Club" because of the address. It was about the best party house in Virginia Beach, and everybody knew about it.

Lila and Melanie were getting ready to go back to school in the fall of '81, and somebody threw it out there that I should just come down to Florida and go to school there. I couldn't get in to the University of Florida, but they told me there was a community college nearby them. "Come on and come live with us and go to school here," Lila said. *Oh, my God, that was such a great idea.*

· 15 ·

THE GAINESVILLE PART

I sprung it on Mom that I was moving to Florida two days before I left. "Oh, by the way, Mom, I'm not going back to school here. I'm moving to Florida and I'm going to go to school there."

She asked how I was going to afford that and I told her I would be sharing expenses with Lila, Melanie, and Janine, and that I would find a job. She didn't want me to go, but there was no telling me not to. Deep down, I always had an adventurous spirit, never afraid of much because, well, it was an adventure!

Once I got settled in Florida, I got a job at a Brew Thru with a gas station attached. The manager was looking for somebody to pump gas. I didn't know anything about cars, but I could sure figure out where the gas tank was. Checking the oil was a whole 'nother story. But of course, I told my boss I could do it. *Oh, sure. I knew how to do all that stuff!*

I remember Jimmy Buffett came through one day. "Can you check my oil?" he said. I was freaking out because I was the only one there. "And fill 'er up, too?" he yelled, as he was walking toward the store. I was like, *Oh, my God, I don't even know where the oil stick is.*

I opened the hood and I was just fucking around, pulling at stuff like I knew what I was doing. Jimmy came out of the store with his package just about the time I was done pumping the gas. He asked if the oil was OK.

"Yes, sir," I lied. He gave me his credit card, which actually said "Jimmy Buffett" on it, so I knew for sure it was him. I don't think I was a parrothead back then, so it didn't really mean a lot to me. I only knew it was Jimmy Buffett, and he was famous. He also didn't get his oil checked.

In fact, NOBODY got their oil checked until I finally asked a friend how to do it. *Fake it 'til you make it!* One of Heather's Rules of Life!

Janine worked at the Brew Thru, too. She knew this really cool guy named Jason who had a red Cadillac convertible. That was around the time of the space shuttle Columbia, which was going to be launched into space and return to Earth for the first time. Jason said we should drive down to Cape Canaveral and watch it go off.

We were all over that idea. *Yeah, let's grab a keg and we'll put it in the trunk!* Melanie said she'd get a watermelon and shoot it full of vodka. Jason always had tons and tons of drugs, so we were set. We got our wine, we got our liquor, we got the keg, and we got some chips because we were getting ready to camp out on the side of the road and watch this space shuttle go off. !!!!ROAD TRIP!!!! We got on the road and arrived in Daytona around midnight.

Jason informed us that it was legal to drive on the beach in Daytona, and he was itchy to do that. I didn't think you were supposed to drive on the beach, but whatever. There we were, top down on the red Cadillac convertible, keg tapped in the back seat, wedged between Melanie and I. We had also "tapped" the watermelon and we were putting straws in, drinkin' it up. We were all fucked up, just absolutely fucked up, hauling ass in a big ol' Cadillac right on Daytona Beach. Next thing you know, there were those flashing blue and red lights behind us, and we were all like, *Shit, shit, shit!!!*

What do we do with the drugs? What are we going to do with all these open containers?

Two officers pulled us over and made us all get out of the car. We could barely stand up, we were so wasted.

"You guys know you're breaking the law, right?" said the taller cop. "No, sir," somebody said.

The shorter cop said, "No vehicles on the beach after dark. Besides that, y'all were speeding," pointing out the obvious. We were just trying to stand upright and be coherent because we were higher than kites.

"You guys been drinking?" asked Tall Cop, checking us all out.

"Yeah, a little. Couple beers," I said. (Meanwhile, there's a whole tapped keg in the back seat.)

Jason started talking belligerent, not a good move. He wasn't making any sense, either. The officer was losing his patience.

Short Cop said, "I need to see what's in the trunk." Jason demanded to know why, and we just wanted Jason to shut up.

"Because it's protocol," said the officer. *Oh, God. We are all fucked. We're going to jail. My mom will be pissed. How will we get out?*

Remember that there was also a bag of drugs in the trunk. We all held our breath, kind of like Hunter S. Thompson, you know, *Fear and Loathing in Las Vegas*. We were shitting bricks.

Somebody volunteered, "It's just a keg in the back seat," but Tall Cop made us take it out of the car. We were praying that would be it, and we were all crowding around the side of the trunk where the drugs were. Short Cop opened the trunk and Janine pretended like she was looking for something. The officer was watching her, getting suspicious.

"What are you looking for?" he asked Janine.

"I'm just trying to get my sweater out of my bag," she said, perfectly straight. I don't know how she did that, but he was convinced.

At the same minute he was telling her to hurry up and find her sweater, I fell down with a thud. Short Cop wheeled around, asking if I was all right. "Yes, sir," I said, jumping up the best I could, trying not to look as drunk as I really was. I just wanted to keep him away from that trunk.

"I guess you've been drinking," he persisted.

"No, shir," I persisted back.

Again: "Have you been drinking?" he asked, getting more annoyed by the second.

"Yesh, shir. I mean no, shir. No shir," I slurred. It was like *Who's On First? What's On Second?*

By now, Short Cop was getting really frustrated and angry. He asked for my license.

I somehow managed to explain that I didn't need one because I wasn't driving. He asked Janine and Lila for theirs. They just shrugged their shoulders. I think they were afraid to try and talk because they would give away how drunk they really were.

"Look, I'm not going to give out any tickets," said Short Cop, under his breath like he was trying not to lose his temper. "Just get the FUCK out of this city NOW and never come back! You are never allowed to be in Daytona again. I'm gonna follow you to the city line. Now, git!"

I had enough of a brain left to know that we were in no shape to drive. *Fuck, fuck, fuck, now what do we do?*

Well, we all got in the car and Jason was trying to drive as soberly as he could, like about ten miles under the speed limit. Tall Cop and Short Cop followed us for about a mile and finally turned off the road. We all breathed a humongous sigh of relief.

Holy shit, can we please just get to Cape Canaveral?

We arrived in the early, early morning, probably like four or five o'clock. Of course, the first thing that comes to my mind is, *Fuck, he made us take the keg out of the back seat! We need more beer.* It didn't even occur to me that we were supposed to return the empty keg that was now God knows where.

It got to be seven o'clock or so, and we pulled over on the interstate. Everybody was parked on the shoulder to see the space shuttle launch. Jason spotted a store across the interstate on the other side of the northbound lanes and Lila and I were nominated to go get the beer.

Carefully, we made our way across the southbound lanes, waiting for a chance to get over the northbound lanes. Lila and I were all chatty, excited about getting some beer, and the next thing you know this car came barreling down on us.

The station wagon hit me in the back and Lila on the side, throwing us both off to the shoulder of the road. *What the fuck??* We were trying to get our bearings and we saw the car keep driving, running right into a parked pickup truck full of tailgaters. They got crushed.

What the fuck just happened? I can't get up. Lila can't get up. Lila managed to ask me if I was all right, but I didn't know. I thought I might have broken my arm or something.

The police came with an ambulance and the EMTs checked us out. We just had scrapes and some bad bruises... it was a miracle. It's pretty ironic because the reason we didn't get seriously hurt is probably because we were so fucked up.

The police officer told us the driver was an elderly man with a plate in his head, and he had blacked out and lost control of the car. The three tailgaters were in critical condition. Another narrow escape.

OK, well, that's over. All good! Now back to the important business of getting the beer, which we did, and rushed back over to the car with it. Jason asked us what took us so long and we explained what happened. They looked at us like, *What the fuck??*

We kicked back in the convertible, just normal life for three college kids on a trip to watch the space shuttle lift off. The launch was one of the most spectacular things ever. It went off without a hitch... we weren't as lucky! All things considered, we dodged a few bullets! Life is one big adventure, isn't it?

After I got settled in Gainesville, my dad and I started talking again. I remember telling him that I was stressed because my rent was due and wasn't sure how I was going to pay it. The job at the Brew Thru didn't pull in a lot of money. I asked him if he would wire me $50.

"Sure, Hooch, I'll send it later today," he promised. I was sooo happy and sooo relieved. I checked my account the next day and damn, the money hadn't been sent. I called him three times before I got him on the phone, when he *promised* he's do it the next morning.

"Okay, Dad, I love you," I said, believing him.

"Love you, too, Hooch." Then I waited. And waited.

It still didn't come, and now I was fucking panicking. I called him again the next day and he picked up the phone after a bunch of rings. I could tell he was drunk. *Shit!*

I said, "DAD! Where's the money?"

In a snarky tone, he said, "Heather, I don't have it, and quit calling me!"

I was devastated. Fuck, I had to borrow rent money from my restaurant manager. In return, I had to go out with him. ICK. I didn't talk to my dad after that.

Sometime later I heard (because I wasn't speaking to my dad) that he had quit drinking and moved into a sober-living community. Evidently, the alcohol really took its toll and was affecting his health. His doctor told him if he ever drank again it could kill him, so I guess he quit.

Eventually I enrolled in the community college in Gainesville. I liked the campus. My three friends all went to the university, so we'd meet at home after school. Melanie was in a sorority, so she was our sorority/fraternity connection. Whenever she went to a sorority party, the rest of us would go along.

That was some crazy, crazy stuff we did at those parties. Man, we did a lot of drinking. We'd also go to places for happy hour where you paid five dollars and got all-you-can-drink-and-eat off the buffet. For us broke-folk, that was perfect.

I never had enough money for groceries. I would get bouillon cubes and make broth, cut up some carrots and put those in there, and pretend like I had vegetable soup. If I had a jar of mayonnaise and a carrot, I would pretend like the mayonnaise was dip. It was tough.

Melanie didn't have that problem, because she came from an affluent family in Norfolk. She and I came from two different spectrums but had one thing in common: we loved to have fun and party our heads off. With her being in the sorority, well, parties just came with the territory. Free beer and liquor, please!!

One time Melanie had to make cookies for her sorority and was worried that she wasn't gonna be able to do it. She called her mom and was like, "How do I do this?" The next day, a FedEx box came, and I'll never forget this because I thought it was so hysterical. Melanie opened the box and I was all nosey about what was in it. (I always loved to see what everybody got whenever care packages came because I never got one.)

There was a letter in there with diagrams on it, step by step, showing Melanie how to make cookies. There were three eggs, some sugar and flour all measured out, a baking pan and some stencils. Her mom was on to something because now people sell meal kits as a business! I thought that was hysterical. *I mean, are you kidding me?*

That weekend we all went to the university to see some bands. I remember seeing Tom Petty. He was from Gainesville, so he played around there all the time. On Sunday afternoons, bands would show up and play for free at the university band shell. You could bring a keg and just sit and listen to the music. I must have played "Won't Back Down" a million times. It was such a blast.

One Halloween, the band was Wendy O and the Plasmatics, an outrageous punk band. If you don't know who she is, Google her. She was a crazy hardcore punker who used to dress up in clear plastic and sing songs with titles like "Living Dead." To be cool, we all decided to dress up like surfboards and go see Wendy O because that's what you did. Of course, we were hammered!

After the show, we found out where she and her band were hanging out, so we went there and drank with them. They didn't know who the fuck we were. But we thought we were "in" because we were with the band, you know? Ha!

It was awesome in Florida, and we had a lot of good times. Sometimes our surfer guy-friends from the 3700 Club would go down to Cocoa Beach to surf, and they'd stop through Gainesville to visit us on their way.

· 16 ·

Russ

Russ and I actually started dating during one of those visits. He was so HOT! Russ went to school at the University of Richmond back up in Virginia. We didn't see each other often, and started writing letters to stay in touch.

I remember I once baked (well, over-baked) some peanut-butter/chocolate-chip cookies and sent them to him at school. They were as hard as fucking rocks. Why I sent them, I have no idea. He told me later that "Those cookies were good, but man, they were hard as rocks. We used them for skeet practice." I was pretty embarrassed, but I thought he was so cute... so cute.

Summer came up fast and we were all stoked to be done with school for the time being. I had kept in touch with Russ and knew I'd see him pretty soon because Lila, Melanie, and I were coming up to stay at the 3700 Club for the summer.

I got a lifeguarding job at the Princeton Country Club. Who gets paid to just have fun? I also started bodyboarding with some guys who invited me to surf with them. I loved being part of the "Dawn Patrol," the bunch of us who went surfing at sunrise. One of the perqs of being the only girl who was in the water with all those guys? I was the ONLY GIRL! I got to see all of the fine asses of the surfer dudes. Always finding positives in a difficult situation! Plus, I got to be near Russ because he was part of the Dawn Patrol, too. Summer was so fun, surfing and bodyboarding and just drinking our faces off.

Summer ended too fast, and we all went back to Gainesville for school. We were still putting on that Freshman 15 even though we were second-year. I look at pictures of us and can't believe how big we were. The Beer Happy Hour Diet!

We got another roommate, a friend of a friend from Virginia Beach. Her name was Taylor. (I can't believe I just remembered that!) She was sort of like the oddball, instead of me. She had some really crazy quirks, like never changing her sheets (gross). She would just put sheets on top of sheets. Her room was a mess. She'd go out horseback-riding and come home and sleep in her bed, and just put another set of sheets on top of the dirty (really DIRTY) set. So Princess-and-the-Pea-ish. Her laundry was creeping two feet out of her door, which was funny because the washing machine was literally right outside her bedroom door.

Anyway, a new school year meant meeting a whole new group of people, like Big Curt (Cute Curt!) from Titusville. He was in some fraternity and his friend, Little Curt, was good friends with Melanie and Lila.

Big Curt and some of his friends liked to do Black Beauties (speed). I didn't know what they were, but they became my favorite thing. *Favorite.* The Black Beauties were awesome because you could stay up longer and drink more over a longer time. I still hadn't tried cocaine because I was too busy drinking and doing speed... thank God for small favors.

I had a massive crush on Big Curt, but I was always just the "fun friend" and he didn't return the attention. I was never the one-night-stand or makeout-in-the-closet-at-a-party type. Kinda sucked. I always met these guys through my girlfriends because nobody was ever coming up to me first. Never good enough, like always. All the girls were a lot prettier than me, and they all had more than me, so in my back of my mind I was always playing catch-up, just like I had for so many years. I was still a dork, drinking my face off. But then all of us were doing that then.

· 17 ·

HURRICANE WARNING

One day we heard from an old high-school friend, Jeff Gadden, who was going to college in New Orleans. It was time for Mardi Gras to come around and he got in touch with Lila.

"Hey, you guys want to go to Mardi Gras?" she asked, all excited. It was a week before exams. I was all in because I think I was just taking one class or two classes, not stressing myself out too much, ha!

And so Janine, Melanie, Lila, and I loaded up Lila's brown Ford Pinto and drove to New Orleans for Mardi Gras. We actually got to Jeff's house without any catastrophes. The first thing he did was announce that we were having some Bloody Marys and then we were going into town. Well, all right!

We had our Bloody Marys and were walking down the street when Jeff started talking about going to this famous oyster house. At that point in my life, I wasn't much of a seafood eater. All I remember is walking by that place, and it had the most hellacious stank. It stunk so bad it was making me sick, but a little nausea never stopped me from wanting to drink some more, so we ended up going to a bar that gave itself credit for being "The Home of the Hurricane," a sweet rum drink that will knock you on your ass.

So we were drinking Hurricanes and taking pictures and drinking more Hurricanes, and then we went down Bourbon Street. We were just plastered, but that was OK because you can drink on the street in the French Quarter. That year the main band was Kool and the Gang (now I'm really dating myself!) They were the hottest thing around when I was in my early twenties.

I remember us going to dinner and me falling over, cutting my foot and losing my shoes. It was a crazy, crazy, crazy night. Eventually we wound up back at the Hurricane bar.

The funny thing about that story is that none of us remember being there earlier in the evening because we were all so wasted. We were all like, *God, these are the best drinks in the world* like it was the first time we ever had a Hurricane. We only found out we were there twice after we got back to Gainesville and got the film developed!

After a long night, we ended up going back to Jeff's house to crash. The following day was Parade Day, which is a big part of Mardi Gras. So we got up and started in on the Bloody Marys again.

We were shitfaced by about ten or eleven o'clock in the morning. Down along the parade route, we found a spot in the bleachers where we could sit, and waited all day for the parade, drinking the whole time. That night, we watched the parade, completely trashed, catching all the beads, with Kool and the Gang playing in the air.

Driving back home in Jeff's VW van, we saw this guy hitchhiking. We stopped at a light, opened the door, and yelled at him to get in. We were all off our tree, just slammed drunk. This guy was a little wary, and so polite, like, "No, it's all right, I'll just wait for a cab," and I said, "No, just get in! We are FUN!!"

That guy probably thought it was a bad idea—it was—but he got in anyway, into the van full of really drunk people. You could see this look of *Oh, my God, what have I done?* on his face.

We were all trying to give him a drink, asking him what he did for a living, slapping him on the back, and being generally rowdy. At that point, he was really rethinking his decision to get in. "Maybe, I'll just go... you need to let me out, okay?" he said, looking kind of scared.

I don't know how he did it, but he jumped out at a stoplight. One of our friends jumped out, too. Somehow, some way, all of a sudden our hitchhiker was upon on the roof of the van, which happened to have a sunroof. Next thing you know, our polite little hitchhiker fell through the sunroof.

"You guys are *fucking crazy*!" he yelled, his politeness gone out the window. "You're gonna kill me. Let me out of here!" So he bolted, and we just laughed our asses off.

We had to get up early the next morning because either Janine (or Lila?) had to get back to take an exam. So we left Jeff's around seven that morning—not before another few rounds of Bloody Marys—driving home in Lila's Ford Pinto. God bless Lila.

We had to make a few stops along the way, like at every fast-food place. People were looking at us like, *Where the fuck are these homeless people from?* We must have looked like we'd been on a bender for about a month, which is pretty much what it felt like. Actually, that was one of my great experiences at the University of Florida. Eventually, though, it came time to get home again.

· 18 ·

BACK TO THE BEACH

After my second school year in Gainesville, I went back to Virginia Beach and lived at the 3700 Club with Lila and Melanie for good. I shared the upstairs with them. We had two small bedrooms, a real small living room, a small kitchen, and a teeny bathroom. The surfer guys still lived downstairs, and now it was gonna be nothin' but a party all the time.

One of those guys was Russ, who I mentioned before. He was my first real love. Blond hair, blue eyes, of course. Another one of the surfer guys actually had a zebra-striped van! They were a trip.

So there I was, back in Virginia Beach. I was lifeguarding part-time, but it wasn't enough money to live on. I heard about a new restaurant that was being built, Graham's on the Water, and I heard that they were hiring. *Why not apply? I waitressed for a couple of minutes before;, I can do it!*

A few of my friends were applying, including Damon, who sometimes rented a room at my Aunt Bonnie's. Just so happens that when they called my aunt's house to schedule an interview with Damon, I was hanging around there and answered the phone. I told the guy Damon wasn't there, and he asked me to leave Damon a message saying Graham's wanted him to come in for an interview. I told the guy that I had applied, too. He asked me for my name and I told him, kind of hijacking the call.

"I'll be the greatest waitress ever!" I lied. "Customers love me. I work really hard!" Well, I got myself an interview and went in to see the manager. I remember this guy named Jim, who had a lot of questions. "Why should we hire you?"

Something came to me that I had seen somewhere, in a book or on TV and it stuck in my head for some reason. I just blurted out, "Because I can be an asset to your business!!" I had no idea what that meant, but it sounded very smart. They hired me on the spot, the first person to be hired for this new place. So I pretty much, again, BS-ed my way in. I'd never really waited on tables except at Magical Pancakes, where I got fired because I couldn't keep up.

Anyway, I was so happy to get hired, so stoked—but also terrified because now I'd gotten myself into this and had to figure all this shit out. There were rules, but not a whole lot, and that's when drinking became really fun. People would get off work and we'd sit at the bar every night and have lots of drinks. We had a namesake drink for the restaurant, the "Graham's Gonzo," which had vodka, gin, rum, tequila... I think maybe a splash of orange juice and some blue Curaçao. You drank two, and you were pretty much on your ass.

The first night Graham's was open was a soft opening, just for the investors. I was so, so nervous, even though I only had a couple of tables. One of my tables was four of the major investors. Why would they put me on that table?? I have no idea. But anywho...

I remember them ordering drinks and I think I got the drinks out to them fine, but when it came time for the dinner, I messed up. Of course, I brought the entrées first and the salad second. They made a joke, like, "Oh, just like we're in France where you get your salad last!" I was still so naïve and probably the worst waitress ever, but Graham's kept giving me a chance. I did get better at it, and it was a fun place to work.

It was the '80s, you know, and I was really into punk and new-wave... Devo, The B52s ("Love Shack" - wow!), The Romantics, The Clash. That was my jam! There were always great punk, rock, and new-wave bands on the strip. If we weren't working or at the beach, we'd be down at Loco's, which was an awesome bar. They used to have shots and beers for like a quarter, and they had the greatest pizza ever.

Eventually, I worked my way up to bartending and even worked the raw bar for a while. I'm sure that's where the term "shucking and jiving" got started, because I'd be shucking oysters and serving beers and I'd have ten people at my bar, laughing and telling them stories. That was a blast.

Lots of drinking, lots of cocaine around... that's the restaurant business. I hadn't done that much cocaine until then, but a lot of people were into it at the restaurant. We had a secret code: "Table 19." If any of us came in hung over, there was a certain manager who would call, "Heather, please come to Table 19" over the PA, which meant you could go to one of the tables way in the back and the manager would lay out a couple of lines of coke to help you get your day started. Way better than a cup of coffee!!

It was a great gig, just the beginning of my illustrious restaurant career. We worked hard and drank hard after work, you know, like-minded people. Even the owner was a partier. Our goals were to have fun and make money, in that order.

It went so well that I decided not to go back to school. I could work nights or days, and then I could go surfing and boogie-boarding. That's what I did in my free time, and even got into competing after a while.

The East Coast Surfing Championship was held in Virginia Beach one year when there were huge, huge waves. I guess nobody else had signed up for the Women's Division and there I was, all ready to go, with nobody to compete against. The officials offered to let me compete in the Junior Men's Division. I went out there and I won! I got this big trophy and five new boogie boards. My mom used to laugh that I won the Junior Men's Division because I ended up beating the boys!

· 19 ·

THE LAST TEMPTATION OF RICHARD

One day in 1983 I got a call at my bartending job. It was my mom.

"You need to come home, Heather," and I rolled my eyes.

"I'm working, Mom, I can't come home." I kept drying the wine glasses and putting them on the rack.

"Honey, I'm sorry to tell you, but your father has died."

I broke down crying, and somebody had to take over my shift. Before I went home, I slammed down a few cocktails, served to me by the person who took over my shift.

I walked in and sat down, only for my mom to wham me again with the news that she and my dad never officially divorced. It was a lot to take in. I found out later that my dad had gone over to my brother Chris' ex's house to see his grandchild, and there was a bottle of vodka sitting on the counter. I guess the "urge" got the best of him. He drank it all and it killed him instantly.

My brothers (except Buff) had left Dad/California a while ago and moved to Virginia Beach to be near our mom. She booked a flight for all of us to go to California for the funeral. What I didn't know was that Chris had left a few outstanding warrants behind in California.

So Mom, me, Chris, and Eric flew back together. My brothers and I were trashed during that whole flight, despite the embarrassment to my mom.

We arrived at my ex-sister in-law's house and all sat in the kitchen for a minute to get our bearings. We weren't there ten minutes and there was a knock at the door. Chris answered it. It was the police, coming after him for those outstanding warrants.

Chris had nowhere to run. The officers barged in, grabbed Chris, and handcuffed him. My mom and I were freaking out. I jumped over the kitchen table, crying hysterically, and slugged the cop. My mom was screaming at me to stop. It was complete mayhem.

They took Chris to jail. My mom had a lot of paperwork to fill out and file, and she couldn't get any real answers about what was going on. It was so frustrating. We were having a small service for my dad, and we tried to get my brother out of jail to attend the service, but they wouldn't let him. I was so traumatized by the whole series of events that I don't hardly remember it, but it left another mark for sure.

· 20 ·

COLLATERAL DAMAGE

At least I had Russ to come back home to in Virginia Beach. He was the first guy I ever slept with. I think we'd been dating for about a year, and I waited *that long* to sleep with him.

About six months after that, I ended up getting pregnant. I couldn't have a kid, that was crazy!! I was only 23, and I was like, *no way*. I told Russ that I probably should have an abortion.

I asked somebody what to do because I didn't know anything about abortions. I learned about this clinic that would do it for like three hundred dollars or something. I asked Russ if he would go with me.

"I think I have to golf that day," he replied. I was like, *What kind of an answer is THAT?*

I was pretty flabbergasted that he wasn't going to go with me. I had no choice but to borrow my Aunt Bonnie's car. I went, I had it done, and I came home. That was it. I was pretty sad.

Every year I'd say to Russ, "You know, if we had kept the baby, it would be this old!" That haunted me for a while. We ended up breaking up but I don't remember why. I think it was probably because I wanted somebody who was going to bring me flowers and do this and do that. Russ treated me very nice, he did—and we had a lot of great adventures together, and were very much in love—but it just didn't work out. The problem was that I didn't want him to have anybody else. I was possessive. Whenever he had a girlfriend, I would always intervene, like go over to his house and see if he wanted a booty call. He and I had this chemistry where we would see each other in a bar, even if one of us was dating somebody else, the feelings were always there. Russ was the love of my life, my first love. We dated for, I think maybe five years in all.

Meanwhile, back at the 3700 Club me and the girls were partying a lot. We were big Elvis Costello fans then, so one afternoon we were sitting around drinking, and we decided we should have an air band because we always used to sing and pretend like we were playing music. So we started our own Elvis Costello air band we called "The Inner

Carrots," and I played the drums. I think Lila was singing, with Janine and Melanie on guitars. I'm sure I'm forgetting somebody... Amy, maybe. What a riot.

We used to follow all of the punk rock bands around and see them play. There was a great band in Virginia Beach called the X-Raves. Kelly Miltier was the lead singer and he was amazing. We were their biggest groupies! They played all these amazing cover songs and some of their own. "Psycho Killer" was one of my favorites, a Talking Heads cover.

I was still working at Graham's, the most happening place down on the beach. That New Year's Eve I worked for the extra holiday pay. My boyfriend at the time, a cop named Gabe, and his brother were hanging out with me, trying to keep up with the drinks I was slamming down. Yep, drinking on the job was becoming the norm for me.

Gabe considered himself a songwriter on the side. He had a Sharpie and was writing lyrics on a cocktail napkin for a song he called "Metamorphosis Is Not Your Name" (LOL). Come time to cash out, I discovered that I had lost my apron full of money. I ended up owing the restaurant like a thousand dollars. It was horrible. I went home, and when I woke up the next morning I had all these crazy words, written with a Sharpie, all over my arms. I guess he ran out of room on the cocktail napkin!

Gabe and I had an argument one night and he stormed out, pissed, and got into his Corvette. He kept a service pistol in his car and was moving it from under his seat and ended up shooting himself in the foot! *Haha, shouldn't have pissed me off, right, Gabe?* That was the end of that boyfriend.

Then I met this guy at work, Tim, one of the bartenders. I had an immediate crush on him. He was the guy who first introduced me to caviar. He taught me how great it was to drink chilled vodka and eat really nice caviar. When I first saw it, I thought, *God, this is so gross.* But I could suffer it because I could always chase it with a shot of vodka.

Tim was also the guy who taught me how to kiss the best. I remember making out with him and he would be like, "No, no, no, you gotta do it this way... No, you got to do it that way." *Oh Lord!*

When I was dating Tim, I was rooming with this guy who used to come to the restaurant all the time. Total preppy guy, car salesman. Nice, but extremely obnoxious. I found out he was looking for a roommate, so I moved in with him. Everybody called him JR, and he had somewhat of a crush on me. My mother loved him. He was like the Eddie Haskell character from *Leave It to Beaver.* All the parents thought he was this real straight guy, but he was pretty much an obnoxious jerk.

Most of the time, my mother was bugging me to go out with him and I was like, *Are you kidding?* The guy was like as white as a milk bottle. I remember he won this ski trip to Vegas and asked me to go with him. I turned him down, but he kept flattering me, telling me how much fun I was to be around. Also so happens he always had a big ol' bag of cocaine, too. I finally gave in.

I didn't know how I was going to do this because the guy was so obnoxious, but I went if for no other reason than it was a free trip and free drugs. So we flew out to Vegas, and during the flight he was so jacked up I was amazed that they didn't stop the plane and throw him off.

We got to the hotel and got our skiing gear. JR had one of those suede-like drawstring bags that we put peppermint schnapps in, and we took some coke with us. We got to the ski resort and JR was like, "Here's how you do it. You do a bump, take a shot of schnapps, and ski down the hill!"

Not the best idea. I repeat: Do not do cocaine and ski down a slope. That was probably one of most horrific experiences of my life. To make things worse, we got stuck on a chairlift. When all of a sudden this massive whiteout storm comes and you are with the most obnoxious guy in the world, you don't want to be stuck on a chairlift. Sometimes, you know, the freebies... you gotta watch what you wish for.

· 21 ·

The First DUI

My first DUI was in Virginia Beach, and that's when I was working at Graham's on the Water. I was seeing this guy named Jaxton Wood. We always said, "Jaxton Wood, if he could." He wanted to take me out to dinner in Norfolk and of course, you know, he liked to drink and drug, too. A match made in heaven!

He said, "Look, I'll get a car (because he didn't have one at the time) and we'll go down to the waterfront district, and we'll go to the Jonas Seafood restaurant (a super-fancy place) and we'll have some drinks and then we'll just, you know, head home, I'll get a baggie and we'll have some fun!" Sounded like a pretty good plan to me.

The night started rough. I think he was late picking me up and there just seemed to be a lot of stuff happening. We got down to the waterfront and parked the car on the street, close to the restaurant. We grabbed a couple of seats at the bar, which was like a long island. It must have been an omen or something, because the bartender told us they were having a special on Long Island Iced Teas in a fishbowl that night (an alcoholic's dream!).

I swear it looked like a gallon of Long Island Iced Tea. I was looking at this amazing, biggest-damn-dream-I've-ever-seen drink, and thinking *game on*. If you don't know what this drink is, it's vodka, rum, tequila, gin, Triple Sec, a wee bit of sour mix, and a splash of Coke (the soft-drink kind). It's a sledgehammer of a drink.

We ordered appetizers, did a little grazing, and chatted with the bartender. We were having a really good time. I ended up having two of those huge drinks. I think Jaxton had one. We decided we probably shouldn't drive, so we had the bartender call a nearby hotel to reserve us a room. We left, stumbling all the way, barely able to walk.

Before we went to the hotel, I wanted to stop and get my sweater out of the car, and Jaxton wanted to get his coke. I got in the driver's side while Jax got in the passenger side to get the baggie out of the glove compartment. That's when the blue lights started flashing. Scared the absolute shit out of me!

We were so drunk we didn't even see the cop car parked right behind us. *Thank God we weren't going to drive!*

The cop got out of the patrol car, banged on the window, and told me to get out. I was scared and didn't know what the hell was going on. I was like, "What did I do, officer?"

He said, "Well, you've been drinking." I said, "Yes, sir." And he said, "But you're behind the wheel of a car, and I'm going to ARREST you for DUI."

I protested loudly. "But the keys are in my hand! I'm not driving!" Jaxon chimed in. "She's not driving! We were just getting our stuff out of the car so we can spend the night at a hotel because we're too drunk to drive!" This was crazy.

"Then why is she in the car?" asked the officer. "Because she's getting her sweater," said Jaxton. The cop was not having any of that, so he gave me a sobriety test, which of course, I failed. He put me in the patrol car and took me to the Norfolk jail!!

I was petrified and crying, and Jaxton was yelling, "Don't take her! Don't take her!" I was scared because Jaxton still had that bag of coke in his pocket. The cop told him if he said one more word, that he'd get arrested, too, and that he better not come down to the station, either. Well, that was no good because I needed him to come down there and get me the hell out of jail.

The cop took me to the precinct, you know, a big-city urban precinct. Lots of lots of black people in there. They put me in this big holding cell with all these people, and they took my shoelaces, which I didn't understand at all.

"Why are you taking my shoelaces?" I demanded, with all these people standing around me, just staring a hole through me.

"Because they're afraid you're gonna hang yourself," one of them said. I assured everyone that I didn't want to hang myself, but they took my shoelaces anyway. Now I was just in there with no shoelaces and a whole bunch of other drunk people. I was scared.

I started yelling. "Why are you putting me in here? Don't I get a phone call? Don't I get one phone call?"

At that point, I didn't even know who to call because I was sure as hell not calling my mother! So I decided to call Sue, a bartender friend. (Sue was always a jokester and we were always playing pranks on each other.)

I finally got to make my phone call, so I called Sue at work.

"Sue, it's Heather. I'm in jail. I need you to come bail me out!" She hung up, thinking it was one of my famous practical jokes. I called back.

"Sue! Don't hang up!" I guess she figured out I was serious, and she said, "What do you mean, you're in jail?"

"I'm in the Norfolk jail for a DUI, but I wasn't driving," I explained. She hung up again.

OK, fine. I called back again and wailed, "I need your ass to *bail me out!!!*" She finally figured out I wasn't kidding and said she'd come and get me.

In the meantime, they gave me a breathalyzer test and I blew a .30. The legal limit is .08. The lady cop said, "Whoa, you're really drunk, aren't ya?"

I started laughing and said, "Yeah, I sure am." She told me that was nothing to laugh at. I didn't get that at the time.

Sue finally showed up and eventually got me home about 3:30 in the morning. Then I had to tell my mom that I had gotten a DUI. You never want a child you love to tell you that.

I had no idea where Jaxton was, so I called him. "What the fuck happened to you?" I demanded, pretty pissed off.

"You heard the cop... he said if I showed up at the jail, I'd be arrested," he said.

I was thinking, *Well, that's great. Our first real date. Not a great start.*

I wasn't really sure what to do next, but I knew I had to go to court, which meant I should probably get a lawyer. So I got a lawyer and told him I wasn't driving and I shouldn't have been arrested, this was so ridiculous, yada yada. He told me he thought he could get me off with maybe doing an ASAP (Alcohol Safety Action Program) class. He did, and I went to the class. It was a few hours long and I was done.

So that was age 24, DUI #1. What I learned: You can pay a lawyer to get you out of your DUI!

PART III
YACHTING CAREER

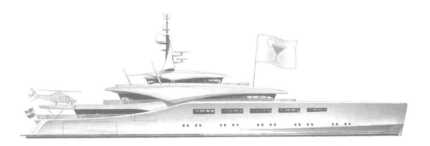

LEARNING THE ROPES

Hobie Cat catamarans gave me my first sailing experiences. Me and my Virginia Beach friends and I would take them out in big weather, more fun that way. I remember one time we were out on a Hobie 16 and the skies got dark and up came a waterspout (basically a tornado on the water). *Oh, SHIT!!* But we survived just fine and I quickly learned that I really liked being out on the water.

There was a boat captain and his first mate who used to come in to Graham's all the time for lunch. Captain Fred and his first-mate Allan were on the motor yacht *Independent Spirit*, a 50-foot boat. They would come in while I was bartending, telling me their tales about the owners, where they were off to, where they'd just been, and such like that. It always sounded like a ton of fun.

One afternoon, Allan came in and I asked him what I could get for him. His answer was not exactly what I expected.

"Have you ever thought about getting into the yachting industry?" he asked. *Huh?* I said I hadn't, and he threw it out there that he and Fred had a really good thing going and maybe I ought to think about it. The families (customers) were awesome and it was a great experience.

He was asking for a reason. "I've taken a job on another yacht and I need someone to take over my duties with Fred. And well, I thought, you know, you're cool, you have a good rapport with customers and you know how to make drinks. And that's pretty much what you would be doing. It's like being a bartender on a yacht."

My ears perked up. *That sounds sooo cool.* "Tell me more about what I would be doing," I said. I was really intrigued by this.

He laid out how I would be putting out a continental breakfast in the morning, serving coffee and orange juice, and then making light *hors d'ouerves* and cocktails at night. Then he told me how much it paid.

WOW. That was a LOT of money for being a glorified bartender!

"You would also help Fred out with the boat," he added.

Gulp. I had practically zero boating experience, but hey, I could fake my way through, just like I did with everything else.

Allan said, "Here's Fred's number. Give him a call, go meet him, and see what he says. Hopefully it'll work for you, and hopefully it'll work out for me."

So I went and chatted with Fred. I actually think he had a little crush on me because he used to flirt with me all the time at the bar. He told me about my duties and stuff. I said "Oh, yeah, oh sure" a bunch of times, like I knew what he was talking about. He asked me if I had ever worked on a boat before, and I had to be straight with him.

"No, but I'm a quick learner and I'm always willing, and open-minded." I couldn't read his face, but I don't think he believed me. "Okay, Heather. Show up on Saturday and we'll go over the boat." *Woohoo!* He gave me a shot at it anyway.

That Saturday, Captain Fred showed me the boat, pointing out do's and don'ts along the way. I was feeling pretty comfortable until we actually took off—or launched, I should say.

"Heather, get the lines off the boat." *OK, what are the lines?*

I guess he figured I didn't know because I wasn't moving. He said, "The ropes," and then I got it. If you're going to be in the industry, you gotta learn the lingo!

We took the boat up the coast to a seaside inn in Virginia where all the yacht owners liked to go. I think we went back and forth a couple of times. Fred did most everything; I just kind of helped him keep up the inside and wash down the boat and stuff.

One of those back-and-forth times we returned to Virginia Beach to the slip where he kept the boat. We had to back into the slip, as in "stern to." I had not done this before, so Fred kept telling me, "All right, Heather, get the port line on." (Port is left; right is starboard.)

Well, I did not know what port and starboard were then, and I didn't want to tell him I didn't know. So he was shouting at me, "Heather, get the port line on! Heather, get the port line on!" And I was like, "I'm doing it!!!" as if I yelled it loud enough it would magically happen.

I was dragging my feet trying to figure it out, thinking *OK, I've got a 50/50 chance of getting it right.* He needed to get that port line on *now.* This was before cell phones, so I couldn't just do a quick Google search to look up how it worked. Fred was getting angrier and finally, I looked up at him and he was frantically pointing to the left.

"Get the goddamn port line on!!" he yelled. I think he wanted to kill me. I learned the difference between "port" and "starboard" the hard way! From then on, I would put I put a green P on my left toe and a red S on my right toe: port left, and starboard right. Whenever Fred would say port or starboard, I would just look at my feet.

· 23 ·

STRANGER DANGER

I did the charter thing on *Independent Spirit* for a summer, until Allan came back. Then I went back to bartending. Probably about six months later, maybe a year, I got a call. "Hey, Heather, this is Allan." *Allan?* "You know, Fred's old first mate?" It had been a while.

"Yeah, sure," I said, happy to hear from him. "How you doing?"

He said, "I'm doing awesome, but I'm in a situation again," and I was wondering what he wanted from me.

He explained that he took a job on an even bigger boat that needed some additional crew, and he wanted to know if I was interested. He went on to say that a little more work was involved because it was a bigger boat. And it was in the Bahamas.

The Bahamas?! That was about all I needed to hear. I didn't care how big the boat was or how much work it was or even how much it paid. All I was thinking about was that I'd never been to the Bahamas! This was going to be amazing!

Allan described the boat a little more and that there would be six guests. I would be charged with making breakfast, lunch, dinner, *hors d'oeuvres* and dessert.

"And oh, by the way, the pay is a lot more than Fred's boat," he said. I was like, *Hell, yeah!!* Just one small detail... I didn't know how to cook. Another chance to fake it 'til I make it!

You haven't heard me talk about a cooking background, you know, because I didn't really have one. My mom was a really good cook and she used to buy all of us kids cookbooks, starting real young. We would take turns cooking dinner. I think I was 10 when we all had to pick out a dinner we wanted to make one night a week. Say Monday night would be my night and I would have to make dinner for everyone, with a little help from my mom, who helped us with the grocery shopping. Every year we all got cookbooks for Christmas, and that was basically the extent of my cooking experience.

Allan told me when I was supposed to start work, and that the captain would be calling me soon. I was going to have to tell my manager at Graham's what was happening and all that. The captain did call, and his name was Robin Walters. That was a nice name, and his voice was really nice and deep. He was very cordial to me and clearly explained everything I would be responsible for. All that was left for me to do was clean up some loose ends, like give my notice at Graham's and tell my mom. So far, so good.

"So, Mom, guess what I'm gonna do?" I said.

She did not like the idea one bit. "You're going off to the *Bahamas*? You don't know anybody there," she said. "You know, you could be kidnapped or something. They drive on the wrong side of the road. Do they even speak English in the Bahamas?"

Oh, my God, Mom, are you kidding?

"Heather, you don't know what you're getting into if you go to the Bahamas. It's full of strangers who could be dangerous. You don't even know anyone to call if you get in trouble!" She was right. I didn't.

I kind of brushed off her protests and asked her for a bunch of recipes I could make on the fly, nothing too complicated. Maybe three dinner recipes, three lunch recipes, how to make pancakes and French toast and I would figure out the rest.

So I flew from Norfolk to Florida and got on one of those seaplanes that lands on the water. I'd never been in a seaplane before, so this was all pretty exciting. I was going to the Bahamas! I was also nervous because the fact was that I *didn't* know anyone there, just like Mom said. I didn't even know how to use the phone over there.

We landed (bumpily) in Nassau, and I was really looking forward to meeting Captain Robin with the Really Nice Deep Voice. I got off the plane and started looking for him. There was a Bahamian guy standing there who was built like a brick house, dressed in a starched white shirt. *Is that my captain? Hmmm. He didn't have a Bahamas accent on the phone.*

Now I was wondering if I crossed signals with Robin. I had very little money in my pocket to get anywhere, so that could be a problem. All of a sudden, the brick-house guy came walking up to me and said, "Are you Heather? I'm Robin Walters." I stood there like a numbnut, not saying a word. This guy was built like a human Transformer, very physically intimidating—and I am not a tiny girl.

Robin must have sensed my uneasiness. He just grinned and said, "Why don't we go get some dinner and just kind of get to know each other?" He broke into a huge smile, and that calmed me down a little.

We went to Tony Roma's, known for its onion-ring loaf and barbecued ribs. I was still jittery because I was really starting to wonder what I was thinking when I agreed to this whole thing. Robin proceeded to tell me what was going to happen on the yacht, and that he would introduce me to the first mate at some point. We didn't hang around long, because he knew I was tired and he wanted to show me the boat before it got too late.

Bedazzled—the name of the boat—was like a 60-footer. (I'm amazed that I can still remember the names of all the boats I was on.) Robin showed me all around the boat, which was huge, and there were just three of us to handle it. *Where was the mate, anyway?*

He said the mate wasn't there. It was already about 10 o'clock at night.

"Let me show you to your cabin," he said. He led me to this cabin that had a twin bed. A little small, but okay.

Robin said, "This is where you'll be staying. I'm going out for a little while, but I'll be back soon. Just, you know, make yourself at home." I thanked him and he left.

I was beat and starting to feel the reality of what I had taken on. It was hitting me like, *Holy shit, how the fuck am I going to pull this off?* My stomach hurt and I was really nervous. I decided to take a walk around the boat and look at the galley (the kitchen, in boat-talk).

I got out my cookbooks and started looking through them, then looked around at the pantry and the equipment and explored the cooking area. Maybe I could do this after all. The guests weren't coming in for a few days, so that was good. That let me relax a little, and I finally laid down to try and get some sleep.

You know, the worst thing you can do when you're anxious about something is turn off the lights and lay in bed awake. Your mind starts going. *I don't know this Robin guy. My mom said it was dangerous here.* I got up and checked the lock on my cabin door again.

After a while, I must have drifted off to sleep but woke up in a panic because I heard the doorknob jiggling. *Someone's trying to get in my room.* They kept trying, trying, trying and I was scared shitless. "Who is that?" I croaked. I think I must have sounded scared because only about half of that came out.

Nobody was saying anything on the other side of the door until I heard a deep voice booming, "Open the door!"

"I'm not opening the door until you tell me what the hell you want!" I yelled, and that time I was mad instead of scared.

The door banged open and some man came barreling into my cabin. It was Robin... in his little BVDs underwear!!

"How do you do?" he said, polite as could be.

"Get the fuck out of my room!" I screamed. *What the fuck are you doing in my room?"* I was up in his face and he just had his underwear on. I was like, *Oh, my God, MY MOM WAS RIGHT.*

I must have said "Get out of my room" five times.

"I'm just checking on you," he said, in that nice, calm, deep voice.

"Get the fuck out of my room," I repeated, and he finally did. Not a really good way to start things off. I slammed and locked the door and started freaking out. I didn't know whether he thought maybe if he came into my room, I'd sleep with him. I didn't know what he was up to.

Maybe I should get the fuck off this boat right now. Should I get the fuck off this boat? I decided to wait about half an hour, put on some clothes, and go up top and take a walk. I got up to the salon—it was pitch black— and I heard this sound, a bumping noise. I jumped out of my skin!!

I turned around and there was this tall, skinny, skinny, skinny black guy standing in the middle of the living room. *HOLY FUCK. NOW WHAT??*

"Who the hell are *you*??" I demanded, looking for the exit. "Who ARE you??"

"My name's Toothpick," he said, all cool and casual.

"What do you want? What do you want?" I was not all cool and casual, and I bolted for the door.

"Wait a minute, wait a minute," he said. "Are you Heather, the new chef?" *Huh? How does he know me? And why was he calling me a chef? I was just a glorified bartender, remember?*

Toothpick said, with a goofy grin from ear to ear, "I'm the first mate."

Oh, my God, Heather, you idiot. He asked me why I was so upset and I told him about the little incident with Robin and his tighty-whities.

"Robin was probably drunk, and was just coming to check on you," said Toothpick, who really did deserve that nickname. I swear I have never seen such a skinny person.

"But he was in his underwear," I said. Toothpick just smiled and said, "Just go to bed. I'll see you in the morning. Don't worry; everything will be okay, you'll be fine."

Right. Don't worry, be happy. Oh, my little brain hurt.

I woke up the next morning and was a little embarrassed because of my reactions—more like overreactions—the night before. But you know, I was in a strange place and these were some strange people.

As I was coming into the galley, I smelled this awful, awful smell. It was horrendous. It was like something died in a pot somewhere in there about a year ago. I walked in and there was Robin and Toothpick and two of their friends with this pot of *whatever* on the kitchen table.

"What is that God-awful smell?" I said.

"It's boiled fish!!" said Robin. "We eat it every morning. Here, try it!"

"Um, no, thank you. No way, no, thank you." I escaped without having to eat bad fish, at least for that morning. I still don't think the smell ever completely got out of my nose.

As the day went along, the crew told me what to expect from this charter group. It was going to be a family of five, and they were bringing their own diving instructor. We were going out for about five days around the Exumas (I had no idea what that was, but it's a district of the Bahamas that's made up of about 165 islands). Toothpick handed me a sheet of paper that listed all the things they wanted to eat and drink.

Toothpick kind of took me under his skinny-ass wing. He took me to the grocery store, showed me what I should get, and told me some good staple-type food to make, things like pigeon peas and rice. He also introduced me to

Washington, the best "Conch Salad" guy in the world. Everybody loves conch salad!! I didn't think I could handle it, but I tried it and loved it because it wasn't fishy. Didn't smell like that awful boiled fish!! Ha! Anyway, I was so glad to get it pre-made because it was totally new to me.

So I got through that first charter, thank God, and had five days to rest until the next one. Everything was good and everybody was like, *Oh, we love your food, we love you.* And I was thinking to myself, *I don't even know what the fuck I'm doing.* But I was doing it, and I was in the Bahamas, the prettiest place I've ever seen in my life. You know, Robin and Toothpick helped me out a lot and it was all good.

The two of them had relatives all over the islands. Everybody knew the Walters family. Robin's brother was Joey, a dockmaster. I used to call him "The egg with legs" because he wore this white button-down captain's shirt and white shorts. His belly was so big and his legs were so short. You get the visual of the "egg with legs!" Joey always had a great big smile on his face.

While I was there, there seemed to be a whole succession of people in Toothpick's family who passed away. One day I came back to the boat and there was Toothpick and a couple of his aunties and a sister or cousin or two... a lot of people. They were all very sad, telling me how so-and-so died and then so-and-so died. In their beliefs, people die in thirteens! They were talking because that day was Number 12 and they needed to think about the funeral celebration because it wouldn't be long before Number 13 passed away.

These celebrations were usually held down near the water, and everyone was welcome, including me. People showed up in the brightest, boldest, most beautiful clothes. It was a large lake-baptism type thing, with lots of music and food. I was so glad I got to experience it.

I swear I thought every single person in the Bahamas was nice. People were very helpful and welcoming and it was easy to get to know the other yachting people (known as "yachties") because the marina where we were based wasn't all that big. I would pick the other chefs' brains and they would give me great ideas.

On one of our charters, I got to learn how to dive in the Exumas. It was spectacular. We were between charters, so I was going to the beach a lot. I'd met a guy who was the captain of another boat, and he knew how to sneak us into the old Club Med resort that used to be there.

One afternoon I came back from the beach to *Bedazzled*, and there was a big red sticker on her. I ran and found Joey (the Egg with Legs) and asked him what was going on with the boat. He said he had just talked to Robin and that the police had seized the boat due to foreclosure! *JOB OVER!*

Robin came down to the marina and said, sadly, "Heather, we are out of a job. I have money for a plane ticket to get you back to Florida."

· 2 4 ·

Yo-Ho-Ho and Too Many Bottles of Rum

What?? I was not ready to leave. I loved that lifestyle. I didn't get kidnapped, and I made some great new friends. But Robin told me I couldn't stay on the boat anymore. *Fuck! What was I supposed to do? Go home? To what?*

I went and found my Club-Med friend and asked him if he might have any work for me. He said he didn't but suggested that I go ask Captain Bluestone of *Breezy*. He might need somebody.

Bluestone was probably in his late 40s, but because of his overboard rum habit, he looked 60. This guy was a champion boozer, way better than me.

(Here is a good place to note that I had kind of promised myself not to drink or do drugs while I was on a boat because I wanted to be responsible, so I had my drinking under much better control in those days.)

I went over to *Breezy* and asked Captain Bluestone for a job. I must have really sounded desperate because he informed me he did have work for me and that I could stay in the crew's quarters. He went through his rules (he was a stern captain) and said that as long as I did my job with a good attitude, there would be no problems.

He taught me so much! Waxing, varnishing, polishing the stainless, and lots more. When our workday was done, I could do what I wanted. (Bluestone usually went to his girlfriend's house.) I guess I proved myself, because the yacht's owner and his wife were coming soon and they needed a chef (there's that word again, LOL). I was offered the job.

The owner was on some sort of Atkins low-carb diet. I remember cooking one egg and three pieces of bacon for his breakfast. His lunch was four pieces of bacon wrapped in a mayo-coated lettuce leaf, along with what is now known as a "Parmesan crisp." Bluestone actually showed me how to make those. I should write another book called *How to Make Your Employer Do Your Job While You Get Paid For It!*

Well, the Bahama charter season eventually came to an end and it was time to take the boat back to marina in Florida. Bluestone, rum in hand, asked me if I wanted to make the trip and work in the boatyard.

"Hell, yeah," I said. My Club-Med friend had given me the name of a woman who owned a yacht-personnel employment agency there. Her name was Sally. I decided to pull my résumé together and go see her.

First, I went to the library and looked at other yacht-chef résumés and put together one of my own that was at least *partly* true. Then I went to the agency to meet Sally.

Boy, was I was intimidated. She told me I needed to do a better job on my résumé. Lucky for me, there was a lady in her office who offered to help me.

Meanwhile, I was working hard in the boatyard and enjoying life. I went into see Sally again and she still didn't have anything, but she recommended that I get up early and go pound the docks looking for work, and to make myself known. I did exactly that.

· 25 ·

LITTLE RASCAL: LOST IN THE SOUP

Sally called not too much later, just in the nick of time, because I was getting low on money.

"Heather, I think I've found you a job. It's a 50-foot sailboat. The captain's name is Mac and he's a real fun guy. Rather large, but very agile. The boat's name is *Little Rascal*. I chuckled. *Oh, what a perfect boat for me.*

"The boat is up in Maryland," she went on. "I'll give Mac your number and he can call you."

He called, and we chatted away. I think he was in a bit of a pinch, and so it didn't take much for him to hire me.

I flew up to Maryland a few days later to meet Captain Mac. Big guy, probably 300 pounds, but agile, just like Sally said. Probably about five-foot-eight or nine. Red hair, red beard. He asked me if had I ever sailed before.

"Of course," I said, which was only half a lie because at least I had been on a yacht—just not a sailboat. I did tell him I was kind of new at it.

"That's OK," he said. "I like teaching. That way you learn the right way instead of the wrong way." I was down with that.

Little Rascal, a full-time charter boat, took four guests. We took people out for five to seven days and that was considered a trip. I remember telling my mom about it, and she was very excited for me.

She said, "Well, I think your Aunt Bonnie and I will drive up there next weekend to see you!" *Hold on, I don't even know if that's allowed,* but before I could get that out, she started telling me about this cute little hotel she booked and about some festival that they wanted to go to. She also wanted to meet Mac, and yada, yada, yada. I think she just wanted to see for herself that I wasn't in mortal danger.

The next weekend rolled around, and Mom and Aunt Bonnie showed up, all excited. I took them down to see the boat and they couldn't believe how big it was. They met Mac, and of course, what's not to love, and so I think that somewhat reassured her brain. At least I was back in the States, and that was better than the Bahamas, in her mind. Good thing she didn't see the blow-up doll Mac he kept on the boat! True, I swear.

The boat was in the yard before the next outing so we could work on it. Mac showed me all kinds of mechanical things and taught me about how the boat was supposed to run, what he expected and everything else. We got along pretty well. I have always gone into a new situation with a willing attitude and an open mind. Just tell me what to do and I will do it. I always wanted to learn and was never a know-it-all... that never worked for me.

Mac and I took the boat up to the Northeast and anchored it in the harbor. First on my to-do list was to haul the laundry onshore and get it done before the next charter. It was a beautiful August day, but up there on the coast, you never know when the fog is going to roll in.

I started up the Boston Whaler (the ship's motorized dinghy) and yelled to Mac that I would be back in a couple of hours. He waved me off and I began to motor into shore, which is only about 100 yards away.

Within a couple of minutes, the fog fell over everything. There was no GPS or boat radio on the Whaler and the fog was getting super-thick, super-fast. I couldn't even see the bow of the dinghy. Everything was dead silent. I cut the motor because I didn't know what direction I was going in, so I just thought, *I'll wait it out.*

I hadn't taken notice of any other boats in the area, but that doesn't mean they weren't there. If there were any other boats, I couldn't see them. I sat there for about 45 minutes and thought I'd start the motor again and just go really, really slow. *Never go faster than how hard you want to hit something*, I always say.

Somewhere in the distance, I heard a rumble, kind of like a boat motor. I started heading toward the sound, going at a crawl. I was tooling around for about 15 minutes, and then I lost the sound, so I started to worry, and besides, it was getting cold. I cut the engine again to try and regroup my brain.

"HEY, is anybody OUT THERE?!" I started yelling my head off.

Crickets. *Fuck.*

I shouted again and again and again. Nothing. There was not much else to do but re-start the engine and putter around some more. At that point, I had no clue how long I had been out there and the temperature was dropping pretty fast. There was an old sheet in the storage seat, so I wrapped it around me and said a little prayer.

Okay, good, someone's listening because I heard the sound of a lobster boat. They have a certain sound; you can tell. I began yelling again, and this time I heard a man's voice yelling back.

"Where are you?" he shouted. I knew this person was really close, so it was funny to hear that.

"I'm right here!!" I was waving my arms, which was dumb because the guy couldn't see me. *Duh.*

The man told me to keep yelling and he would follow the sound of my voice. I told him I was lost and had no idea where I was. His boat slowly came out of the fog (I was right; it was a lobster boat) and the captain asked me where I was headed.

I was pretty embarrassed to say I was just heading for the marina. *How do you get lost on a 100-yard trip?*

Then he asked, "Which marina?" *What? What do you mean, 'Which marina?'*

I told him the one in the north harbor and he looked pretty surprised. He pointed to his right and told me if I went that way that I'd find land. Apparently he was going to leave me on my own to find my way back.

"Girl, you were on your way out to the Atlantic," he said. Just as I was ready to start freaking out, the fog cleared. I asked him what time it was, and I figured I had been floating around for about four hours. That nice man escorted me back to *Little Rascal* with my dirty laundry, where Mac was waiting to greet me.

"Where the hell have you been?!" he roared. He was not a happy camper, and the laundry still hadn't gotten done. It was all too much and I just started bawling my head off.

"But I've been lost at sea! The fog came in! I got turned around!" I wailed. It was all very dramatic, but I guess it worked because Mac forgave me. I never got in the dinghy again without a radio!!

· 26 ·

LITTLE RASCAL: THE HOITY-TOITIES

The sailing vessel *Little Rascal* turned out to be a pretty good adventure. We were now in North Harbor, setting sail to South Harbor to pick up a seven-day charter, this time a group of four. I learned that the primary guests were from one of America's richest families. I'll call them Tom and Laura Moneybags. Son of a bitch, they were rich! They brought another couple with them, Jared Moore (a famous vineyard owner), and his wife.

Of course, you have to stock up the boat before you leave. You make a grocery list, only it's called a provisions sheet. For this charter, the provisions sheet kept getting changed back and forth because Laura kept going back and forth about what she wanted. She seemed a little high-maintenance.

Come to find out that Mrs. Moneybags had put her husband on a diet without him knowing it. No cheese, no butter, no carbs. There were a couple of things she definitely did not want on the boat, and one of those things was lobster. I guess because they lived in the northeast, they got enough of it. *(Who cares about what their guests might like? LOL).*

Everybody was safely boarded, and we were off, heading to some little island they owned, somewhere back up around North Harbor. On the third day, Laura came down to the galley and said, "Heather, we would like a lunch of steamed lobster with drawn butter, corn on the cob, and some dessert. We would like it packed up and we will take it to the island with us."

None of these things were on the provisions sheet, because it was a NO-FUCKING-CARBS and NO-FUCKING-LOBSTER CRUISE, remember? ARGGHHH! *Yeah, right, so you think I could just whip that up?*

And I was like, "Well, I didn't get any lobsters." She got kind of huffy and snarky and said, "Well, I'm sure you can find some." Then she added, "Oh, yes, and make that a blueberry pie for dessert."

I rarely, rarely bought blueberries. One, because I just didn't use them that much. Two, because they stain—countertops, carpet, cloth napkins, chair cushions. Messy little things.

I told Captain Mac we needed to find some lobsters. We actually flagged down a lobster boat that afternoon and a bought them right off the boat. Lucky. And for some weird reason, I had gotten a thing of blueberries for that trip. I was like, okay, so I'll make the pie. I made their beautiful little lunch, packed up a picnic basket and sent them on their way for their little outing on their little island.

The Vineyard People brought this really nice cheese and they wanted me to put it out for *hors d'oeuvres* that night. I arranged a nice little platter of cheeses and meats, you know, *charcuterie*. As Tom Moneybags was going in to get some cheese, Mrs. Moneybags slapped his hand, saying, "You can't have that. You can't have that."

He was like, "Why not?" And she said, "Because it's not on your diet."

Tom snapped, "*What* diet?" She loudly explained how she had told him he needed to stop eating dairy, fat, and carbs. A pretty feisty argument ensued and they went back and forth, back and forth... very uncomfortable for all aboard.

The next day we were sailing from Point A to Point B and Mr. Moneybags decided he wanted to play captain and sail the boat. Mac said it was OK. Meanwhile, I was down below, making soup for lunch.

Mac was on the bow, watching the fog, thick as pea soup. We had to go very, very slow. My soup (not pea) was in the microwave while I was downstairs looking at the LORAN (short for Long Range Navigation System – most people call it a fish-finder). Tom was on the wheel and Mac was way up on the bow, trying to see ahead into the fog—that's how thick it was. Well, I heard Mac start yelling at Tom, "Go port, go port, turn, turn!!!!"

THUD-CRACK! We hit an underwater rock. Mac was hanging off the bow rail, because we hit so hard, it had flung him over the rail! Like I said, he was very agile, so he was able to pull himself back up onto the boat. Me, I had soup all over my galley, leaking out of the microwave, everywhere. It was just a big messy, sticky fiasco.

All in all, those people were just a pain in the ass for the whole trip. Plus, they smelled like mothballs. *Maybe mothballs smell like old money, huh?* Ha, I don't know. But after a week-long charter (that felt like three weeks), we finally were dropping them off and they were saying what a wonderful, amazing time they had. By then, Mac and I were thinking to ourselves, *Get the fuck off this boat and out of our sight.*

The Moneybags handed Mac a tip check for the trip. Usually when people charter a boat for a week and it's just two people, usually we'll get a tip of, you know, $300, $500. This was four people, so we were thinking, maybe $1,000. Mac opened the envelope and I could read his face, which said, *What the hell is this??* and I was wondered why his face looked like that. The Moneybags had lots of dough, lots of it. But Mac's face was oh-my-God, and not in a good way. He showed me the check. It was for $150.

I was sooo pissed. I worked my ass off for that charter and all they tipped us was $150, after telling us how great everything was. On top of that, they crashed the boat!! I told Mac to give it back to them, that it was insulting. Then I thought maybe we should cash it and leave a nasty note on the back! I was just so pissed off. Mac couldn't believe it, either.

One last thing: When we dropped off The Moneybags, the matriarch of the family was there to greet them, one very famous lady. I met her. Back then, it didn't mean anything to me; people were just people and that was it. But I think it's pretty cool now. *Wish I could tell you who it was!*

· 2 7 ·

THE FLOATING CLOROX® BOTTLE

After my adventures on *Little Rascal*, I was hired on to the "floating Clorox bottle," which was named *Vinda*. It was a sailboat, a motor-sail 70-foot Bristol. If you look that up, you'll see they're very round, very roll-y, just like a bleach bottle. Instead of gliding through the sea, it rolled back and forth. Luckily, I didn't get seasick back then.

Vinda took me all the way to the Virgin Islands. It was the first time I ever did a delivery, and that was pretty cool. The captain, Nick, was a real big drunk, and he wasn't the nicest drunk either, so that made things... interesting.

Just before we left, I ran into a couple of my friends from the yachting industry at a resort bar, and was telling them that my captain said we were leaving on Saturday. (That was on Friday afternoon.) We were chatting away, and the mate Henry showed up and announced that the boat was leaving. Not Saturday. Right that minute. *Excuse me?*

Henry explained that we were leaving for the Virgins that night but didn't say why. I was kind of freaking out, and for good reason. Nick had been at the same bar, drinking away all afternoon. Not good for a captain about to sail a ship.

So I had to make a big decision: Do I stay, or do I go? I didn't want to let the agency down that hired me, but I didn't want to do the equivalent of getting in a car with a drunk driver, either. My gut was telling me *NO!* but the job was telling me *YES!* I wanted more jobs from the agency and might not get them if I bailed at the last minute. I decided to go. My friend gave me her St. Christopher's necklace and told me to wear it for protection.

I was really scared, and pissed off, too. How could Nick be so irresponsible and get so drunk? I left the bar around 8 o'clock, just so nervous about getting on that boat, but I did.

I didn't have a watch shift for a while, so I put on my bright orange life jacket, went down to the master state room, and just laid there in the middle of the bed, praying. We had been underway for maybe around 40 minutes, and all of a sudden, I heard—and felt—a big crash. Crunch. *Crunch.* THUMP. Squeeeal. And the boat came to a complete stop.

I was like, *Oh, my God, I'm going to die. I'm going to drown.* I ran upstairs. *What the hell?* Well, we had run aground. Hit something. I don't remember if we hit the reef or just ran aground.

A sea tow came to pull the boat free, which took about three hours. They hauled us back to Florida and had divers look at the boat hull the next day. Repairs were done, and I think we left in a couple of days after that. I also think the captain may have learned a lesson, and that was not to drink all day and then take the wheel.

Light winds at the outset of the trip back left us in the what they call "the doldrums" for about four days. That was fine with me after all the initial excitement. The rest of that charter was nothing more than a long, uneventful trip, thank God.

We anchored back in the Virgins and were met by the owner, who was with a guy I remembered meeting somewhere else, on one of my other boats. His (not-real) name was Ed Richilieu, but I think you'd know his real name. A very wealthy guy, big on the horse circuit. He was, I think, like a billionaire. One of the rudest men I've ever met in my life. I remember Captain Nick telling me that this bigwig guy was only going to be on the boat for a couple of days and that everything had to be to the "T." He was very fussy and demanding and was going to want this and that when he wanted it. I was like, *OK, no problem.*

Well, the first hour the guy was on the boat he managed to insult me twice within the span of 30 seconds. Nick didn't tell me he was a complete asshole.

"Girl, where are your tits? Why don't you have any tits?" He was like almost taunting me. Then he looked over at the captain and said, "Why would you hire an unattractive chef with no tits?"

Oh, my God. I thought Henry, the mate, was gonna tackle the guy. I walked upstairs and right off the boat! Henry came running after me, all the way down the length of the dock, begging me to stay. I told him I couldn't stand being around that jerk and that I was just going to take a walk, go up to the bar, get a drink, cool off, and then come back. I kept telling myself that The Bigwig Asshole would only be on board for one more day. I could hold my nose for that long.

I eventually left *Raj.* It was a headache all around, but one good thing came out of it, and that was that I met (what I thought then) was the love of my life! He was a young Mel Gibson look-alike. First guy I ever met who literally left me speechless. More about him a little later.

· 28 ·

SEX TOYS & THE ART OF CLIMBING PALM TREES

My next vessel, the sailboat *Privilege,* was one of my favorite boats to work on. It was an 80-foot custom pilot house ketch that could take six to eight people. The crew of this boat is what made it special.

Captain Stan and the first mate Paulo were both ex-Navy SEALs. My friend Lauren was the stewardess, and then there was me, the chef. We were based in the British Virgin Islands, which was a blast. I called it the "milk run" because we usually picked up guests from one island and then sailed over to another island to clear customs.

Our first stop was Jost Van Dyke, one of the smallest of the islands. Back in '88, it wasn't nearly as populated as it is now, so it was a lot easier to navigate. We would anchor off a really famous bar there called the Soggy Dollar. The bartender, who I'll call Kip, was this really good-looking Bahamian. Kip made everybody feel special, and he loved us because we brought passengers in who tipped a lot. We tipped a lot, too. This was a serious hangout for charter industry people, and we all helped each other out.

One really cool thing the Soggy Dollar had was a big chalkboard. You could write the name of another charter boat on the board, pre-pay for a round of drinks, and sign your own boat's name... then when that charter came in to anchor, they'd see on the chalkboard that they'd have a free round of drinks from *Privilege* waiting for them! *How cool is that?*

We had a couple of really interesting charters on that boat. For instance, there was a couple from New York, and we could see from the minute they walked down the dock that they had "high-maintenance" written all over them. They had lots—*lots*—of luggage. As soon as we set sail, the complaining began.

"Oh, my God. It's too sunny here. Aren't there any clouds? Oh, my God, there's too much sun. Is it gonna be this hot the whole time? Oh, is it going to smell like sea water?" The wife would not shut up. Everything was an offense to her dainty little self. That sort of set the tone for the trip.

We set off and took them to the Soggy Dollar for our first stop. The next day, we might go to Foxy's restaurant. They usually had a band, and you could call ahead and pre-order dinner. They would ask what you wanted: Chicken, fish, whatever, depending on what they had. We would ask the guests for their choice. We'd get there and tell them we had a reservation for *Privilege*, and they'd bring us dinner. Chicken or fish, with pigeon peas and rice, a nice salad. It was awesome.

Nobody had cell phones then, so I always had to call Foxy's using the VHF radio and identify my boat and my "handle," like truckers do. My handle was "Fallen Angel." Ha!

One of the days on the High Maintenance trip was really windy. We were sailing south, tacking left and right—port and starboard, I should say—and all of a sudden we heard Paulo (the first mate) just cracking up laughing. He came up from down below, still laughing, trying to contain himself. He managed to say, "Heather, I need to see you in the galley!"

Usually before we left, we always double-checked to make sure the portholes were closed tight. Everything that might break was put away/stowed because we were gonna be heeling over to port, heeling over to starboard, rocking back and forth. So I was thinking, *Shit, we didn't check the portholes.*

I went down below and Paolo said, "Heather, you need to go look in the port cabin."

I expected the worst. "OK, so there's water everywhere, right?"

Paulo said, "Nope. Go look."

I went into the port cabin and saw that one of the drawers had fallen out. What I saw in that drawer is something I kind of wish I would not ever see again. It was a bunch of super-kinky sex toys, like three dildos and some double-ended thing with lots of wires and stuff on it.

Oh, my God, I thought. These people were the prissiest, most fussy, doom-and-gloom people in the world, and they had all these wild sex toys on the boat. I mean, the boat was 80 feet long, but did they think we wouldn't hear something?

I was laughing hysterically and called up to the captain, saying "Stan, I think I need you down here." He came down and saw the drawer, and then HE lost it. I went up top, took the wheel from Lauren, and told her to go check on my lunch stuff. She went down below and Paulo told her to go look at the port cabin. Now everyone was cracking up. That became our humongous, hilarious secret on *Privilege.*

After that little incident, we made a game of constantly looking to see who had, you know, bright, rosy cheeks. Ha! The best part was at the end of the charter. The couple was getting ready to disembark, and Lauren and I were handing the luggage to Captain Stan and Paolo, who set one of the suitcases down on the dock. It immediately started vibrating.

The couple was like, "We have to go, we have to go!" They were mortified. I just asked, "What's making that noise?" and we all started to laugh. All they could say was "Thank you for a great trip!" as they ran down the dock, and all we could yell was, "No, thank YOU!!" That little episode made my whole week. It was just hysterically funny.

People are sure different. Take the Tanager family from the West Coast. They used to charter quite a bit with us. Julius Tanager had a bunch of fast-food franchises up and down the state, along with an alpaca ranch and an avocado farm. Julius' wife, Louisa, was really nice. Very outgoing and just very pleasant. Their daughter, Kate, went to an Ivy League school. They had money to burn.

On one trip, Kate brought her boyfriend, so there were four of them. Lots and lots of drinking, those people. I remember us going to Peter Island (one of the little out-islands), which was known back then for their Mudslide ice-cream drinks. You had two, and you were pretty much off your tree.

We anchored, and the guests got off the boat right away. We stayed behind for a little bit to secure the boat and clean up, then we would usually meet the guests for happy hour. Sometimes I'd stay behind to finish preparing some amazing fish dish or something (!). By that time, everybody was pretty well lit.

After dinner, they all wanted to go back up to the bar, and they were begging me to go with them. I thought, *What's a few drinks?*

So we all went up to the bar, and we were getting looser and looser and looser. At some point, I found myself sitting on the beach with Paolo and Kate. I noticed that Paolo was chatting up Kate pretty good. Julius had gone back to the boat. Louisa and Captain Stan were sitting in lounge chairs by the pool. The boyfriend was nowhere to be found.

Well, after five Mudslides and wine with dinner, I was feeling no pain. I also thought I was 10 feet tall and bulletproof, so why not do a barefoot climb up a palm tree?

"Hey, watch me!" I yelled, and started up the tree. I got halfway up and thought, *This is hard. Why do my feet hurt so bad? How am I going to get down if my feet hurt?*

I didn't wait to figure it out and just started sliding down, scraping the hell out of my knees on the very rough trunk. The bottom of my feet were bleeding. It was horrible. The moral of that story is don't climb palm trees while drunk and barefoot, especially when you're not a climber.

I'm sure a lot of other shenanigans ensued that night. The proof was my pounding head the next day, which was on fire from drinking all those sweet drinks. Ouch. The first thing I realized is that I had to get breakfast going. *But wait, I'm not in my room. Oh shit.*

It was one of those really, really bad moments when you're afraid to open your other eye to see whose room you're in, and who's next to you. Well, I looked over and it was Kate's boyfriend. I was like, *Fuck.*

After I had three seconds to wake up, I looked around some more and saw that at least I had all my clothes on and I was on the right boat.

"What happened last night?" I asked, still half-slurring my words. My bedmate giggled. "Not much," he said. All I could think was that I had to get out of there. "Please, no one can know this." Stan would have killed me and I never could have explained it.

I tiptoed over to the door and peeked out to make sure nobody was up yet. It was about seven o'clock, still early. I rushed to my cabin, brushed my teeth, washed my face, and changed my clothes. I felt like dog shit.

Where's the Diet Coke? I need a Diet Coke before I can even think about making breakfast. I found one and chugged it in an effort to make myself feel somewhat better. I had decided to make Eggs Benedict, and put out a really nice fruit platter with fresh pastries and such.

As I was making this lovely breakfast, everybody was slowly coming out of their cabins. At least I wasn't the only one feeling like dog-doo. I announced that Eggs Benedict was coming, and they were all happy.

Then I heard, "Heather, can I get a mimosa?" Then, "Hey, Heather, can I get a Bloody Mary?" *Are you kidding me, you want to drink some more??*

Well, they're the guests, so I started handing out Bloody Marys and mimosas. I downed a few myself and started to feel halfway normal. I served them this magnificent breakfast. Everybody was happy and full and got up from the table, leaving me with a "boatload" of dishes to do. Lauren started handing them to me, and all I could think was, *I am totally not up for this.*

Normally, I would throw any uneaten fruit out the porthole to feed the fish and stuff. But *this* morning, I couldn't be bothered with cleaning sticky egg and cheese and bacon grease off the plates, so I was throwing everything out the porthole. If I could have, I would thrown the plates out too, because I did not feel like doing the damn dishes.

I was thinking, *Hey, I'm being pretty smart and efficient right now* until I heard Stan yelling from up on deck.

"Heather, get your ass up here!!" *What did I do?* The list of possibilities was long. I was sure he had found out I was in the cabin with a guest. *Oh God, please get me out of this.* I climbed up the stairs.

"Heather, what the hell are you doing?" he said. I must have looked confused.

"I'm just doing the dishes," I said, so innocently. He told me to look over the side of the boat.

The boat's dinghy was tied up smack under the galley porthole, and I had just chucked a whole bunch of breakfast food right into it. It looked like a horror egg party.

The sight of that made me start throwing up over the side, and Captain Stan could only remind me that now I had a second mess to clean up. *Worst day ever!*

· 29 ·

PRIVILEGE: THE CHINESE FIRE DRILL

We were doing a cruise through the Caribbean with six guests (three couples). They were nice, fun-loving partiers, but they started drinking early: Bloody Marys in the morning, and tequila shots as soon as the clock struck noon.

A lot of the time, the crew would drink with the guests. Always just good fun and not considered inappropriate at all in the boating world. We were doing just that and ran out of ice, so I alerted Captain Stan. No problem, he would just run the dinghy over to Foxy's and execute a little resupply mission.

Thurmond (the main charter guest) and Lauren decided to go with Stan. I was working on that evening's dinner, so I stayed behind. What happened next would always haunt me.

The trio was approaching Foxy's, just fooling around and having a good time. Lauren and Thurmond thought they would do a Chinese fire drill; you know, you're in a car, you get out at a stoplight, run around the car, and get back in before the light changes. In this case, they were in a 16-foot Boston Whaler dinghy instead of a car. Crazy Thurmond and Lauren actually JUMPED OUT into the water. Stan started yelling, "WHAT THE HELL?" and Lauren was screaming for help. Stan had *WTF* all over his face, and he stopped the boat, shouting, "Where are you, where are you!"

He ran to the back of the boat and saw that the line had wrapped around Lauren's neck and around the prop. The prop was getting ready to slice her throat.

Stan cut the power to the boat and jumped in to free her from the rope line. Lauren was pretty banged up, but he got her back into the dinghy. She started screaming, "Where's Thurmond? Where's Thurmond?" She was yelling at the top of her lungs but wasn't getting it out very well because she was in such shock.

We were wondering where Thurmond was, too. *Shit. Where was he?* Stan jumped back in the water and dove down. (He was an ex-Navy SEAL, remember.) He was coming up, going down, coming up again. Still no Thurmond.

Now the people on the dock were wondering what the heck was going on. Stan went down, came up again and said, "I can't find him." Then other people started diving in, trying to find Thurmond. This went on for about 20 minutes until they finally found him, lying on the bottom.

It turned out that when he jumped out of the boat, the prop knocked him in the head and left him unconscious, and he drowned.

I could hear a lot of chatter on the VHF radio while I was cooking in the galley. People were talking about something happening over at Foxy's. *What?* I heard Stan yelling, "Get Paolo, get him over here! Get him over here!" I asked what was going on and he just yelled at me to get Paolo over there.

I kept trying to get Paolo, who was still at the Soggy Dollar. Finally, I got hold of him and told him something was wrong and that I couldn't help because I was stranded on *Privilege*. The others had taken the dinghy out; I was stuck. Paolo managed to borrow a dinghy from someone at the bar, and he sped over to get me. We hauled ass over to Foxy's. *Where was Stan?* I was looking all over and didn't see him. *Where was Lauren? And Thurmond?*

Someone on the dock said they were up at the Blue House. (If you've ever been to the Caribbean, you know that the buildings are named after the color they're painted. The Pink House is the store. The Yellow House is the school. The Blue House is the police station. And so on.)

We hustled up to The Blue House. I saw Stan, and he was so distraught, just beside himself, bawling. I had never seen him like that, not ever.

"What happened?" I cried, "and where is Lauren? Thurmond?" I was thinking that something really bad might have happened because they were all pretty buzzed when they left. *Shit.*

Stan looked at me with blank eyes and told me about Thurmond, and said Lauren was upstairs in the bathroom. By that time, I was pretty hysterical. I ran upstairs, and there she was, a shell of the girl I knew. The bubbly, fun boat stewardess, sitting on the side of the bathtub, rocking back and forth, her skin color like ashes. Her eyes were so distant.

Lauren wouldn't look up, and even though she was sitting right there, I felt like I couldn't find her. I kept saying, "It's Heather, it's Heather!" I put my arms around her and asked her over and over if she was okay. I saw the marks on her neck from the rope line. It was horrible. And horrifying. We sat there for the longest time, just trying to settle out the shock.

Meanwhile, the other charter guests (including Thurmond's wife) were still over at the bar. We realized that we had to figure out what the heck to do, because Thurmond had *died*.

"We need to go over to the bar and get his wife, Heather," said Stan. "You take Lauren and go back to the boat. Get her in her bunk. I'll deal with the Mrs."

Can you imagine that? Being on vacation in paradise, and some freak accident like that happens on the second day of your trip? One minute your loved one is there; the next minute, he's gone.

Eventually, everyone made it back to *Privilege*. I was just trying to cope and do my best. All I know is to feed people, get them wine, make people comfortable. It was so hard... there was such a very sad, heavy blanket of emotions over the boat.

We weren't allowed to leave the harbor until there was an investigation. All those poor people wanted to do was just go home. Thurmond's wife had to deal with getting his body shipped back, not an easy thing when you're in another country. The authorities wouldn't even release it until the investigation was completed. That poor woman.

There was a formal inquiry, and thankfully, Stan was found not guilty. The whole thing was crazy, one of the worst experiences of my life. It took a long time for Lauren to deal with that, and honestly, I don't know if you EVER really get over something like that. I never did.

· 3 0 ·

THE ICEMAN

All boat chefs use a "provisioner," somebody you can call and order your food from for the next charter. It's like a personal grocery shopper.

Julie, who ran a place called Charter Cuisine in the Virgin Islands, was the lady I always used there, and she was awesome. Julie was like a little spitball of fire, and she pretty much taught me everything, because as I told you, I really didn't know a lot about cooking. Whatever I was reading in *Gourmet* or *Coastal Living* magazine was what I was doing.

The first time I ordered from Julie, she promised my groceries would be delivered the following afternoon, adding that she would include a little "surprise" for me. Because my boat was out on the hook (out in the harbor at anchor), the delivery would have to be made by boat.

So the next day, I was piddling in the galley or something, and the mate called me.

"Heather! Your groceries are here. You need to come up and get them!" he yelled.

I kinda blew him off and said, "Just get them for me, will ya?"

He was pretty insistent. "Heather, NO, you really need to get up here and get your groceries!"

I climbed up top, and at the stern of the boat I saw this guy standing there. I walked up to him, and he said, "Hi, I'm Andy!"

My jaw dropped, and then I just froze in place. Andy was the hottest guy I'd ever seen in my entire life. Sandy brown hair. Crystal blue eyes. The biggest smile! He kind of reminded me of a young Mel Gibson. I'd never seen anybody so hot, EVER! I was starstruck and dumbstruck and all kinds of struck.

"How you doing?" he asked, all sexy and shit.

I just stood there staring at him, like an idiot, and then I ran downstairs! I didn't even get my groceries. The mate was shouting at me to get back up there, but I was petrified. I didn't know what to do. *This guy was so hot... oh my God. Do I hide? Do I go up?* I went upstairs and apologized.

"I'm sorry about that. My name's Heather." My face was as red as the sunset.

Andy said Julie had told him all about me, and he smiled his big, gorgeous smile again.

"Oh, she did, huh?" I wondered just exactly what the hell Julie had told him. "Did she tell you that I was crazy and didn't know how to speak?"

He just laughed it off and handed me the groceries. "Let me know if you need some ice, because I also deliver that out to the harbor."

I sure did take note of that, and thanked him politely. He headed for his delivery dinghy and shouted, "I'll see you soon!" and roared away.

The mate—an amazing sailor, fun guy and great friend—was still standing on the deck, and I turned to look at him.

"THAT is the best-looking guy I have ever seen," I said, practically drooling. "I think I'm in love." My friend just laughed and shook his head.

The next day, I was in Julie's store, telling her that I had gotten her "surprise" and she started laughing out loud. I told her what I had told the mate: that Andy was the hottest guy I'd ever seen in my life.

"Yeah, he's cute all right. And he's *single*," said Julie.

I couldn't believe it. "That guy? Oh, my God. He's so hot. But there's not a chance in hell he's going to like me." I must have repeated how hot Andy was about 14 times. Julie looked at me like I had lost my mind.

Not too long after that, I ran into Andy again and he said, "Hey, I'm taking my boat out. Going sailing on Sunday, if you want to go. There's a bunch of us going." *Dreams really do come true.*

I knew I didn't have to work that day, so I said, "Well, sure! Where am I going to meet you?" He told me to come down to the dock around ten o'clock in the morning, and to bring whatever I wanted to drink. He'd have food and everything. Well, I came to find out that Andy was also a chef—actually one of the better chefs in the entire yachting industry.

Off we went, setting sail on the Hottest-Guy-Ever's boat. I met a bunch of his friends, but still felt like a third wheel. I was so insecure, just trying to fit in like always, you know. I was so transfixed by that guy I nearly forgot my nervousness. It turned out to be a really great day.

When it came time to leave, Andy suggested we go get a drink and have a little something to eat. *Who was I to say no?* We meandered into town, had a drink, and just chatted. Then I went home, just flat-out smitten with this guy, my mind racing with what might come next.

Now I had to play this waiting game. *Did he like me? Was he going to ask me out again?* He hadn't called me yet. He must hate me. I don't know. *Ack!!*

I saw him around town a little bit, and he was still delivering my groceries. We started flirting, and it gave me that nice, tingly feeling I loved to feel. We started to see each other, and that's about the time I got on to my next boat.

This one was an 80-footer, still in the Virgin Islands, just further north. Andy was working another boat in the same general area. I remember that he was going out for this prestigious cooking competition with some other charter-boat chefs. He had a great idea for a dish: Cornish game hens stuffed with a whole fresh mango that was marinated in Grand Marnier. Then he planned to reduce the pan juices to make the sauce. Wow.

That's one of the recipes I remember most from my yachting career. It was phenomenal, served on a bed of risotto with just some simple, fresh vegetables alongside. He ended up winning with that recipe. Actually, I think that competition was sponsored by Grand Marnier. That liqueur was one of my favorite things in the world to drink!!

Andy didn't seem to drink a lot, or at least not anywhere near as much as I did. My drinking was more under control since I started the yachting thing; I still drank a lot, but not like when I was going to school. You had to stay pretty disciplined to work on a boat, and I worked hard at doing that.

Whenever I was off work, however, me and the crew would go up to Sollozzo's, an Italian restaurant that was right up the road from Andy's house. Local place, good bar, awesome drinks. They always had nice Champagne and really good food. A perfect place to spend all my hard-earned money.

Another friend of mine always had a little bit of cocaine, so we would meet at Sollozzo's and do some lines and hang out in that bar all night. In those days, I was spending a lot of my free time up in the north end of the island. Some people might have phrased it more like "Andy-stalking," ha!

I would stay over up there on the north end sometimes, and Andy would have to drive me back and forth. Sometimes I'd get a taxi, but that could get pretty expensive.

One day he asked me why I didn't have a car, and I guessed out loud that it was because I didn't want to spend the money. He mentioned a friend who had a car for sale and offered to help me fix it up. So I bought this awesome Suzuki Samurai (Jeep-like, but not an actual Jeep). Andy put big tires on it, so it was really, really fancy.

A pretty good deal for Andy, too. On the first day of a seven-day charter, he'd walk me down to the boat and kiss me goodbye. I'd hand him my keys and he'd use the Samurai all week. Meanwhile, I would pine away for him while I was gone. *Geez, I was sooo ate up with him!*

Jimmy Buffett's song, "Grapefruit – Juicy Fruit" would always come on the radio while I was away, and I'd always get sad and wish Andy was right there with me.

Every trip, on the last day, I'd be like, *Can't wait to see him, can't wait to see him!* Very slowly, I started moving stuff into Andy's house. You know, a few dresses in his closet. Toothbrush in the bathroom, this and that. I thought I was really sneaky and smart. He never asked me to move in, but I figured he was driving my Samurai, so this must be *something*.

People would ask me to do stuff with them, and if I hadn't heard from Andy, I would make excuses not to go do stuff because I thought Andy would call. I was so ATE UP with him. Every action I took was based on his availability and what he wanted. I didn't make a move without considering him first, so much so that it got to be a pretty unhealthy relationship on my part, and probably his, too.

Sometimes I look back and think it was convenient for him. I really never thought I was good enough for him. I was always thinking there were all these pretty girls around, and he was probably really looking at them—not me. *So insecure and co-dependent!*

One night we were watching TV and Andy jumped up and said, "I gotta go see Mateo," and I offered to go along. Mateo always had the coke. "No, no, no," he said. "I need you to just stay here and I'll be back in a few hours." "Here" was Andy's little one-bedroom place, like a mother-in-law house. He took care of the big house down the hill below him.

So I resigned myself to watching some TV alone. While I was doing that, Andy and Mateo were busy doing something else, who knows what. Andy didn't come home until way late that night. I fell asleep on the couch.

Around two a.m., he came blustering through the door, all out of breath. "You're not going to believe this, and you can't tell anybody!" he said. "You can't tell ANYbody, OK?"

I said OK, half-asleep and not knowing what I was saying "OK" to.

Andy was talking really fast, telling me how he and Mateo found two *bales* of cocaine out near one of the little islands. He was right; I didn't believe it.

"Here, take this!" he said, and a shoved a bag full of coke into my hand.

"What? You found this? Well, that's awesome, thanks!" and I just put it away. Back then I was doing cocaine just for fun, on the weekends—and not every weekend, either. I wasn't addicted (yet) so it wasn't a problem to just stash it for some other time.

That was my life then: partying and partying some more up at Andy's, then I'd get my provisions, clean my galley, and go off for a week. That went on for a while and our relationship was just sailing along, big pun intended.

When we were back on shore, Lauren and I still hung out in the bars with the other "yachties." We got nicknamed "The Tilt-a-Whirl Sisters" because we were so crazy. She and I would go downtown and hit as many bars as we could in one night. There were so much fun to be had, and there were many times when she and I would do a little baggie of coke and go dance on the bar tops and leave at four o'clock in the morning. Just too much fun.

At that hour, there are all kinds of people out lurking around in the shadows. Sometimes I'd see this like six-foot-five Rasta dude. The guy always creeped me out because he always seemed to just be around, waiting for something. Parts of the downtown area were known for some bad elements. I always thought, *STALKER! KILLER!* or whatever, and he worried me.

One afternoon, Andy and I were at the car wash, which was really a drug-deal place. Everybody knew what you meant when you said you were "going to the car wash."

Except this time, we really were going to wash the Samurai because it was muddy as hell, and all of a sudden, the six-foot-five Creepy Rasta Dude came up and said, "Hey, Iceman." (That's what the locals called Andy because he delivered ice in the harbor.)

Andy smiled and said, "Hey, how ya doing?" and I was like, "You *know* that guy??"

Andy explained that he was "kind of a friend, you might say." Rasta Dude looked down at me and said, "I know who you are." That scared me because I'd only seen him in the shadows at night. He and Andy looked at each other with a secret nod. I found out later that he knew I was the Iceman's girlfriend.

After that, Rasta Dude kept an eye out for me and Lauren. How 'bout that, I had my own Rasta bodyguard!

It was September of 1989, and Hurricane Hugo was getting ready to hit. Captain Stan gave me the option of staying in St. Thomas with Andy or going with him on *Privilege* down to Culebra, Puerto Rico, one of the biggest "hurricane holes" in the Caribbean. That might sound funny if you're thinking a hurricane hole is a place that tends to have hurricanes, but it's actually a kind of safe haven where boats can safely hide out during a storm.

"You've got two hours to decide," he said. It took me all of one second to say, "I'm staying." Andy was ruling my decisions then.

And so Captain Stan took Lauren and Paolo and sailed *Privilege* to Puerto Rico. I stayed with Andy at his house, along with my friends Miranda and Jack, who came over to ride the storm out with us. Their house directly faced the spot where Hugo was supposed to make landfall. All we could do was pray that their house wasn't going to get demolished. It was getting pretty scary. I say when you're scared, have some drinks! Lots of them!

Miranda used to love her rum and Coke, so I used to call her "dumb and choke" because that's how she ordered them when she was drunk. She was a very beautiful, exotic girl and I was always jealous of her and of her friendship with Andy—even though she was married to Jack.

The storm was really coming on, and when it finally hit, it was frightening. We had pulled all the mattresses in the house into the living room and were hunkered down on the floor behind them.

The noise is what I remember most. It was so very loud. The cement walls of the living room were swaying in and out, in and out. We were so scared, laying on the floor, praying, praying, praying. Then there was no sound at all. Crickets. Eerie.

"Is it over? Is it over?" Somebody kept saying that. I said it in my own head. Andy got up and opened the front door, and we all looked outside. Everything was dead still, no sound, no movement. No birds. No geckos. It looked like there had been an apocalypse. Everything was torn down: trees, houses, everything just thrown around like a junkpile. It was awful.

Andy stopped and said, "Oh, my God, wait, we're in the EYE of the hurricane right now. We need to get back inside, like now!" We all raced back in and braced ourselves for the back side of the storm.

Just like they say, it sounded like a freight train that was coming right for the house. *We are gone*, I thought. *This is it. I'm going to be buried alive in the rubble.* But I was with the man I loved, so that would have been OK, crazy as that seems.

The hurricane lasted for hours, but it seemed like forever. Finally, there was no sound again.

We went outside and it was so much worse than the first round. So much worse. We couldn't see any houses because they weren't standing anymore. The house below us—the one Andy took care of—was a shredded mess. The top half was ruined; the bottom half looked somewhat salvageable. If you looked at the top, you could see their toilet and the bathtub. Luckily, the owners weren't there.

No electricity, no power anywhere. Jack's business partner came up and the five of us made camp down the hill in what was left of the big house. There was a propane grill and a big playroom-type area, so it made sense to camp out there. We had no way to cook anything or boil any water up at Andy's.

Everyone had their chores. We took turns hiking up the mountain to find water so we could cook and take a shower. (Yay for solar power, because the solar shower gave us hot water!) We had to manually fill the toilet tank with water so it could be flushed.

After three days of this, everybody was going little nutty. Jack and Miranda were finally able to make their way through the debris-filled roads back to their house, only to find it totally gone. It was horrible. They came back to our house because they had nowhere else to go.

I remember getting in touch with my friend Alyssa, who said she had ice, which might as well have been diamonds. Ice was a real commodity because it was hot as hell. I went over to Alyssa's and got some ice and a generator, too. While I was there, I asked if she had any rum (why not?). Making liquor a priority in the aftermath of a hurricane should have been a serious clue that I was becoming mighty dependent on alcohol.

We were doing pretty well at surviving. Andy really knew how to live off the land. He knew landscaping, and he knew about trees. There were trees down everywhere, so he got his machete out and he and Jack started opening up the fallen palm trees. There are hearts of palm in there, a real delicacy. They come in a can at the grocery store and are damned expensive. Here we had them for free, as much as we wanted. We had hearts of palm for breakfast, lunch, and dinner.

Thank God for the gas grill. Without power, it's all we had to cook with. I learned to make a lot of stuff on that gas grill and we ate surprisingly well.

After a couple of days, I started worrying about Lauren, and whether she made it to Puerto Rico okay. I got on the VHF radio and asked if anybody had any eyes on the sailing vessel *Privilege* over in Puerto Rico? Radio silence, as they say. Not a word.

On the third day, there was a response. Somebody said, yes, there were three people on the boat. I borrowed a little cruiser and headed down there to check on everything. I pulled into the harbor and saw nothing but boats—like 50-foot sport-fishing boats—all piled on top of each other. There were boats on top of houses, boats way up on the beach, boats up in the trees. It was like some giant picked up all of these toys and just scattered them around. It was the weirdest, most crazy thing I have ever seen. That's how wicked this Hurricane Hugo was.

Finally, I found *Privilege* and I saw Paolo and Lauren, who were both in this kind of daze. There was no fresh water, so they were just drinking rum. It was hot as fuck and they couldn't shower. The boat smelled like shit because the food had all gone bad. Stan said the only thing they could do was clean her up in hopes that she could go back into charter service. There was nothing I could do, so I went back to the Virgins and back to Andy.

How was I going to pay my bills? My boat and my job were toast. I think I worked a little bit with Julie in the provisioning business, but then I heard that Regus Bay was looking for waitresses. Regus Bay has one of the most beautiful beaches in the world, and they have great beach bars there. That meant I could wear my bikini and make money at the same time!

By then I had a lot of experience, so it was easy to get the job. That was the good part. The not-good part was when Andy and I started having problems.

I started noticing things like money being missing. I had bought a really nice camera that went missing. Andy made me feel like maybe I just misplaced it. *Of course, I had misplaced it; you're right.* Because I was so co-dependent in that relationship, I would never make waves, no matter what. Even the crappy stuff—I would just push it under, like an ostrich with her head in the sand, oblivious to what was going on around me. Lots of denial, just to stay with that beautiful man.

I even overlooked the fact that for the first six months of the relationship, he smoked crack. *Oh, did I forget to mention that?* I was so in lust with that guy, I looked right past it. One day I came home from work and Andy was sitting there on the couch. He asked me if I wanted to get high. He had this pipe and put some foil and something on it, handed it to me, and told me to smoke it. He said it was cocaine. *Why would I smoke it and not snort it?* He told me to just do it and it would be the best buzz I'd ever had.

Again, anything to please that guy. I took a hard hit off of that thing and got the best adrenaline rush I've ever experienced in my life. If you've ever been to a carnival, you know they have those things where you take the big mallet and slam it down and it sends the thing up to the top to hit the bell? Well that's what it felt like to me.

Then Andy told me it was crack. *CRACK!!* I had never smoked crack in my life. But I have to say, I was at the top of that bell thing, at Number 10. Once you're there, you want to stay there; you don't want to come down to Number 7, so you want another hit. I did, and the second I did that I said to myself, *This is the most addictive thing I've ever put in my body, and I can't do this again.*

I put it down and said it out loud: "I can't do that anymore, really, I can't." But

Andy was like, "Oh, but you can!" He kept smoking and I noticed he was getting just fucking weird and trippy, even scary—really paranoid. I took off that night and came back the next day, hoping he'd be "normal" again.

He was on the couch again when I came back. I sat down, gave him a kiss, and we picked up a previous conversation where we had been talking about going to the Rose Court restaurant for dinner.

He turned to me and out of nowhere, he said, "This isn't working for me. You need to move your stuff out and we need to not see each other anymore."

What the fucking hell? I was in total shock. TOTAL shock.

"What is it, what is it, what did I *do*??" I was begging with my voice, taking the blame for something I may or may not have done! Panic started setting in. I was devastated, so unbelievably devastated. I didn't have a boat to live on; I'd been living with this guy, and my friends were always saying, *you're so ATE UP with him*, you need to focus on something else. But I was so crazy about him and the thought of being without him was scaring me into this big panic.

He just said, "It's not working out for me. But I tell you what, let's at least have one last dinner and go down to the Rose Court anyway." Sap that I was, I said okay. *Zero self-respect.*

We went to dinner and it was just stupid little conversation, and we went home. He "let" me sleep at the house, but the next morning he told me to start getting my stuff out and to ask Julie if I could stay with her.

It so happened that Julie had an extra room, so I pleaded with her to let me move in there. I was just fucking devastated, my heart ripped out of my chest. But at least I had a job in Regus Bay and I still had my Samurai. It was so typical "me" to be all sunny and positive in such a shitty situation. I was great at denial.

· 31 ·

THE ICEMAN COMETH BACK

Sometimes I would wander down to the marina, just to walk around and check out the boats that were docked. There was this boat called *Aquabella* and I met the chef, Tina. She was really nice. Her first mate, Mickey, was kind of cute. We all started hanging out, having drinks and stuff. It was good because it kept my mind off Andy.

After that, I'd go home to Julie's and we'd have wine. I had to stop going out so much because I was so broke at that point, just trying to make a living and pay my rent.

Put that on top of being so sad about Andy, and it was not a good time. But then I finally got done with being sad and started making friends at my waitress job down at Regus Bay. I was making nice money on the beach, and I looked good. It was fun, and I started getting my confidence back. I had started a whole new life.

The day after my 29ᵗʰ birthday I was still working down on the beach. I was just doing my thing, and who should walk up but Andy, right out of the blue.

He said, "Heather, can I talk to you?" I'm like, "No, I'm working," just as bitchy as I could.

He persisted. "But I really need to talk to you."

"I am working," I shot back. "You can't be here when I'm working." He asked me what time I got off work and I told him six o'clock. He asked if he could meet me at Julie's house.

"OK, if you really feel the need," I said, all sarcastic and everything. I waited until 6:45 to leave and finally go home, just to be a bitch. He was sitting on the porch, waiting, and never said anything about me being late. I felt all that raw heartache come rushing back. At the exact same second, I thought, *GOD! I nearly forgot how fucking cute he was, so easy on the eyes.*

"What do you want, Andy?" I unlocked the door and we went inside.

He said, "I just wanted to bring you a birthday present." Well, I lost it.

"What?" I yelled, not holding one thing back. "Why the fuck would you bring me a birthday present? We are not together. Why are you doing this to me?" I was getting really angry.

Andy handed me a little velvet bag and I opened it. It was the same necklace Miranda had, a pretty gold chain. I was always telling Andy how much I admired it because it laid flat on her neck, and in the sun it would sparkle.

"This is gorgeous," I said, melting a little. He asked me if I loved it.

"Yes," I answered, "but how am I supposed to feel about this?" I hated that he had done that. "Yeah, this is pretty. But you could have at least gotten me the fucking matching bracelet!" He looked at me like I was nuts.

I told him to just get the hell out of my house. He said, "But I want to talk to you about working things out."

And I was like, "We ARE NOT working anything out."

I was sure about that because Andy had been smoking a lot of crack and he was really going downhill. He had moved into this pretty cool Japanese-y house. There were a couple of parties there that I ended up at... a whole different group of skeevy people. Andy was losing weight and getting more withdrawn, and was not the outgoing, confident guy I used to know.

And so Andy got put away on my Old Boyfriend shelf, at least for the time being. Then it was just me and Julie.

Julie didn't have a washing machine, which meant I had to take my clothes down the mountain to the laundromat. In the Virgin Islands, you drive on the left, not the right, like you do in America. It took some getting used to. Coming down the mountain, there are a couple of really, really tight turns, and one little place where a big rock juts out of the mountain and you have to be careful.

So I was driving and singing along with the radio, about 10 o'clock in the morning. I had gone out the night before, but came home at a decent hour, so I was feeling pretty good, awake and everything. Just singing away and not paying attention, and I came to the damn jutting rock and hit it with my front wheel.

The Samurai was thrown up an embankment and start rolling over, and over, and over. It finally stopped and I landed in the back seat, on top of my laundry, which probably saved my life. *God, what just happened?*

To this day, I remember feeling like I was in a fucking clothes dryer, just tumbling and tumbling in such slow motion. I was screaming because of the crunching of the windows. I was thinking for sure, *I'm dead.*

Then there was a voice saying, "Are you OK? Are you OK?" Some strangers pulled me out and asked if they could go home and call somebody. (No cell phones then, just landlines.) The only number I could remember was Andy's, and so I rattled it off. I was really out of it.

The ambulance came, and they brought a stretcher. I was still a little ways down the incline from the ambulance, and the strangers were helping me walk up the street to get to it. Well, the EMT guys forgot to lock the brake on the stretcher, and I heard somebody shout, "WATCH OUT!!"

Next thing you know, the stretcher barreled into me, knocking me down. Everyone was like, "Oh my God oh my God oh my *God!*" and everyone was telling everyone else to help me up. My neck and back were already shitty from the car accident, and now they were a lot worse.

Andy showed up and started yelling, "Are you okay, Noodle?" (That's what he used to call me.) "Are you OK?" He must have said it five times. Or even ten.

I didn't know how I felt. The EMTs were putting me on the stretcher, locking my head down, locking my arms down because they didn't know what was up with my back or my neck. They got me into the ambulance, and Andy said he would meet me at the hospital, which was about ten minutes away.

The ambulance started going down the mountain, and I swear I smelled burning rubber. I thought I was having a stroke or hallucination or something until I heard the guys up front cussing, "Shit, shit, shit, *shit!*" The brakes had gone out.

The driver was trying to control the ambulance with the emergency brake. They were able to get to the hospital parking lot, gliding in, and the driver finally pulled the emergency brake all the way. That's how we got down that mountain. All I could do was say, "Thank God, thank God."

Some guy rolled me into the emergency room and Andy was waiting there. I was in so much fucking pain. He started screaming at all the nurses, "Get this, get that, get this girl some pain pills, give her a shot, something!!!"

He called Julie, and she was there almost instantly. She thought I was dead; I wasn't, I was just badly banged up, but I guess I looked so bad that I shouldn't have been alive. The hospital released me late that afternoon, but the doctor said I shouldn't even try to walk for at least three days. The fact that I didn't break anything was a miracle in itself. That was quite a day. Another time I lived to tell the story!

Julie took me back up to her house, and there they were, Julie and Andy taking care of me. How dysfunctional is that?

After I healed up, life got back to normal pretty quickly. Andy dropped out of the picture again, and I was still waitressing down on the beach, living at Julie's. Julie was an awesome person to live with, but she didn't want anybody messing in her space. I can understand that now, but at the time I wasn't the most respectful roommate.

There were times when Julie would go to work, and *whoops*, I would be out of cocaine so I'd snoop around for some of hers. She wasn't stupid; she kept that shit hidden from me. I was also never supposed to drink her wine. Boundaries, ha! That was just Julie.

She came home one night to find me with a friend I hadn't seen since I lived in Florida. He'd come into town, and he and I stayed up all night out on her deck, doing blow and drinking. I think back on it now, and yeah, it was fun, but that was so disrespectful. It hurts my heart, the things I did, always disrespecting and hurting my peeps, and not even realizing the damage I was doing.

Anyway, after the mountain accident and the birthday-necklace mess with Andy, I started hanging out with Mickey, the cute mate from the *Aquabella*. He was hot, but he was arrogant, and he was just another one who had pretty blue eyes. There I was again going, *Oh, he's so cute, who cares what a jerk he is*. Mickey treated me like shit, so of course, I liked him.

I remember being in bed with him one time, and his phone rang. We were in the middle of me being below his waist, if you know what I mean. He picked up the phone and started having this conversation. This is when I had one of those glimpses in life where it hit me: I have no self-respect. I was laying there with this asshole who didn't even like me enough to pay attention to me while we were having sex. The feeling of shame crossed my mind, and it's hard to remember that without wincing. It's even harder to write it. (That feeling is what I would come to call "The Ick.")

By the time I was 30, my yachting experiences had taken me all over the Caribbean, and I really started getting my foot in the door. The last couple of years in the Virgins had been good ones, but it was time for a change, so I made my way back to Florida.

· 32 ·

CAPTAIN SAM & FEEDING THE BIGWIGS

I got a call about a yacht charter in New York. Good news: a great potential gig. Bad news: anxiety, insecurities, feeling like an imposter, all bubbling up again. New York people were a lot more demanding and uptight, and I felt a lot more self-conscious around them. I was always afraid I was going to be found out, that people would discover that I didn't really know what the hell I was doing.

But I went to New York anyway, and met Captain Sam and his wife, Allie, who used to be the boat's chef. *Redux* was a really cool sailboat, a 76-foot Sparkman & Stephens racing boat, with a collapsible hull. You could take the settee sail out after lunch and you'd be left with just the skeleton of the boat so the owner could race it.

This couple had a pretty extensive racing "program," as it's called. It's like an itinerary. I remember Allie explaining how it worked, with all the destinations and schedules and lunches and racing. She also told me how my first meal was to be done, including what to serve and even how to do the place settings. She was big on details.

Captain Sam laid out how he ran his boat. He seemed very strict and very much like a "my way or the highway" kind of captain. That all made me really nervous, because these people were very professional, whereas my other boats were kind of roll-with-it.

So there I was, on a new boat with a new crew that was extremely TOP-NOTCH. I was so nervous. No room for mistakes, and that made my anxiety level pretty high. The first hurdle was to work with Allie on an "important lunch for some really important people," according to her. And I was thinking, *OK, important, got it. But I'm just cooking the food. And it's just lunch. And they're just there for the day. I can do this.*

Allie and I were going over the menu and she suggested that it might be nice to have an elegant lunch, like some poached salmon. For dessert, something light like a blueberry mousse. She asked me if I knew how to make that, so, of course, I told her I knew how to make blueberry mousse.

Oh, my God. The only mousse I ever knew how to make was to mix some berries with Cool Whip and stick it in the freezer.

Saying I could do it was a wrong, wrong thing to say because I didn't know what the fuck I was doing. I tried to make the mousse and it didn't set. It's called *Cool Whip* for a reason, and it's going to melt when you take it out of the fridge, right?

Allie saw the unholy mess and said in a real stern voice, "Heather, this is a very important meal. GET IT TOGETHER." I had to confess that I didn't know how. She ended up making the mousse for me because I had to focus on the rest of the meal. *Ugh. The imposter got called out.*

The guests began arriving, one by one. Well, I'm not on the Wall Street circuit; I'm just, you know, this girl from Virginia Beach who's doing the best she can. I found out that the people who owned the boat were big business people. BIG people. Billionaire #1 was a TV big shot. Billionaire #2 was a tech big shot. The other billionaire was a media big shot.

You would know all their names. In the end, they were just people coming out to a sailboat for lunch, right? I at least had the sense not to eavesdrop or start a conversation with any of them because I was so afraid of messing up. There was probably some good gossip to be heard!

In the end, I just winged it. I'm amazed that I did not have a panic attack and just pass out. I was making the crew nervous and I'm sure they were second-guessing their decision to hire me, wondering whether I could do this job or not. But I pulled it off! Still shaking my head over that one, but damn, that lunch was good. (Recipes for the salmon and the mousse are on the next page.)

You know, each boat I worked on gave me the chance to learn something new, including *Redux*. When we weren't sailing, we had to do maintenance on the boat. Everybody did. Like I said, Captain Sam was very strict about the way he liked things done; he was a perfectionist almost to the point of being a bit of a dick, but learning all of that stuff really helped to get me a foothold in the business.

I always knew that if you were willing and open-minded, people would be more apt to teach you stuff. If you're afraid and say you can't, they won't. A friend of mine taught me that "can't means won't." Whenever I would say, "I can't do this," he would look at me and say, "Can't means won't, Heather! Don't be a victim!" So I tried and I learned and I got better.

POACHED SALMON WITH CUMIN RAITA

Ingredients for the salmon:
3 cups dry white wine
1 small onion, sliced
3 celery ribs, chopped
1 T. whole black peppercorns
3 parsley sprigs
One 3-lb. fillet salmon, skinned and pin bones removed
6 thin lemon slices, for garnish
12 thin cucumber slices, for garnish

Ingredients for the Cumin Raita:
2 cups plain Greek yogurt
1/3 cup finely diced and seeded cucumber
1/4 cup finely diced red onion
1 garlic clove, minced
2 T. fresh lime juice
3 T. minced capers
3 T. minced cilantro
3 T. minced dill
1 T. ground cumin
Kosher salt and freshly ground black pepper

Directions for the salmon: In a fish poacher or pot large enough to hold the salmon, combine the wine, onion, celery, peppercorns, and parsley. Add 3 inches of water and bring to a boil. Add the salmon fillet, fully submerged, and bring the liquid back to a simmer. Cover and simmer very gently over low heat until the salmon is just cooked through, about 8-9 minutes. Turn off the heat and let fish stand for 5 minutes.

Using 2 spatulas, carefully transfer the salmon fillet to a large platter. Dab off any white bits and let stand at room temperature for 15 minutes. Cover loosely with plastic wrap and refrigerate until chilled.

Directions for the Cumin Raita: In a medium bowl, combine all of the ingredients and mix well. Chill thoroughly.

Garnish the salmon with the lemon and cucumber slices, and serve with the raita.

Serves 10-12.

HEATHER'S FUCKED-UP FROZEN BLUEBERRY MOUSSE

If you want to feel fancy, go ahead and make this recipe, but I'm sticking with my original version of the mousse!

Ingredients for the mousse:
4 cups fresh blueberries, divided
1 can (14 oz.) sweetened condensed milk
1/4 cup fresh lemon juice
1 8-oz. tub Cool Whip topping, divided
Edible flowers for garnish

Line a 9x5-inch loaf pan with foil, with ends of foil hanging over sides of pan. Mash 2 cups of the blueberries in a large bowl. Add the sweetened condensed milk, lemon juice, and 2 cups of the whipped topping; mix well. Pour into prepared pan. Cover with ends of foil. Freeze 6 hours or until firm.

When ready to serve, invert the dessert onto a serving plate. Remove the pan and foil liner. Spread on the remaining Cool Whip, top with remaining whole blueberries, and garnish with edible flowers.

———⊙⊙———

I remember Sam giving me a project to do, which I did. I went up to him and said, "Hey, Sam, I finished the project." He looked at me like I had just called him an asshole! Daggers in his eyes. I was looking around as if I had missed something.

He yelled, "If you ever say that you're 'finished' again, I'm going to FIRE YOU!!"

Then he explained that there's *always* something to be done on a boat. You start at the stern, and you work your way to the bow. When you finish the bow, the stern needs to be done again. The work is *never* finished. This boat had a lot of varnished areas, so that made sense. All I could think was, *Geez, this dude is intense!* But I got what he was saying.

The first leg of the program was to take the boat to the Virgin Islands from New York. We had a crew of five, and my main job was to prep the boat and cook for the crew, but that wasn't hard. The day we left, there was snow on the deck of the boat! In all, it was an uneventful trip, and we safely got to the islands. There was just one thing.

We were about halfway there, and it was my turn to stand watch and steer. It was dark and I had to look out for the buoys and boats and stuff. Captain Sam showed me and said, "You see that light? Head for that." and I thought I did. Well, I didn't. That was the first time I figured out that I was nearsighted. You should never lie about seeing a light because you could take the boat way off course or hit something. From then on, I kept binoculars on the whole time and looked through them every five minutes. Amazingly enough, I didn't hit anything on that watch. Thank God. (I did get my eyes checked when we got back.)

We dropped anchor near the island where I had spent the previous couple of years. Lauren was still there. My life was just 9-to-5, working on *Redux*. I got to be good friends with the first mate, Kyle. He irritated me on the trip over because he was just as perfectionistic as the captain. It's probably why the captain hired him. I just didn't like all that strictness; I'm like, just get the shit done and have fun doing it. You're allowed to smile, right? I actually had a captain once who told me and my stewardess that we weren't allowed to laugh anymore because we were too loud. I was like, *Just exactly how far is your head up your ass?*

Anyway, that job on *Redux* lasted for a while and then it was over, but that wouldn't be the last of me seeing the Captain Sam.

· 33 ·

DYSFUNCTION JUNCTION: HIM AGAIN

Let's go back for a minute. About a month before I left New York on the racing sailboat, a few friends had called me from the Virgins. They were worried about Andy (my crackhead ex).

They kept calling me and calling me and finally I talked to one of them. I avoided the calls because I didn't want to be reminded of him.

"Heather, you need to go back to the Virgins. Andy is not doing well."

Umm, he's not my boyfriend anymore. Yeah, they said, but he's killing himself; he's like holed up in a closet. I guess he was just really cracked out and his friends thought that I was the only one who could get through to him.

I still cared for him, of course, but I was on a new boat and had a commitment. I told them I would be heading back to the islands in about a month, and that was the best I could do. I promised I would try to call Andy in the meantime.

By that time, Andy had moved into the Japanese house. I heard stories about how he would just start having these paranoia attacks. He wasn't going to work. He was just hiding out in a coat closet and deteriorating. It did worry me.

The first thing I did when I landed back in the Virgins was to go see him. I barely recognized the Hottest Guy Ever. It was heartbreaking to see him that way.

"Andy, you need to get some help," I said, stating the really-obvious. "You're killing yourself." There was so much pity in my voice and I felt so sorry for him. But he wasn't having it. "I'm fine," he said.

"Well, you don't look fine," I argued, thinking about how cute he used to be. His appearance had changed so much. He wasn't that hot, hot guy who left me speechless when I first met him. He was becoming a skeleton of a man and just looked sickly and unhealthy.

I talked to Julie about it and she didn't know what to do, either. We thought maybe an intervention or something, but by that time, I had to get back to my boat.

Some months later, I found myself back in the Virgins again, just delivering a boat back to its home base. I remember calling Andy to see how he was. He sounded better and asked if I wanted to have dinner. While he was talking, I stopped listening and started thinking, *Hmmm... hot ex-boyfriend and I'm just in port, you know. "Any port in a storm" lol? Maybe I would get a little somethin'-somethin'.*

We met at a Mexican restaurant and I ordered a margarita. He got a club soda.

"Aren't you going to have a margarita?" I asked, getting real curious all of a sudden. He said he wasn't drinking and smoking crack anymore, and that's why he wanted to see me.

"I'm four months clean," he said. What a great surprise! "You said I was killing myself, so I got clean." *Well, how about that?*

He went on. "It's part of my sobriety that I have to make amends." I didn't really know what that meant, but I told him to go ahead while I started on my third margarita.

"You know, you talked about how I treated you. I'm sorry for that." He told me about stuff he had done. "I took your camera, your money, and the other things."

Wow! So I wasn't crazy. I thought I had just lost all of that stuff.

"I was sick. The other thing..." He hesitated for a like a whole minute, leaving me to wonder what the hell was going on. It felt like he was going to drop a bomb, and he did.

"In my AA meetings, they tell me I have to change the people I hang out with, the places I go, the things I do. You know, I'm not going to really be able to be in touch with you for a while."

"Why? What did I do?" My eyes started tearing up.

"It's not about you," he said. "It's about me starting over."

Ummm, okay. So does that mean we were not going to sleep together tonight? That was what I was focused on, because by then I was pretty buzzed. *I wanted a piece of that!*

So instead I said, "Okay, I wish you well then," not really grasping what was happening. We finished our dinner and he went home. I probably went to the bar.

· 3 4 ·

FALLEN ANGEL

I found myself back in Florida after the Big Andy Kiss-Off, looking for my next gig. With the most perfect timing, my old mate Henry from the *Vinda* called me from Antigua, in the West Indies.

"Heather," he said, all excited. "You should come down here. Lots of hot guys. You could probably find some work down here!"

He offered to let me stay on the boat he was taking care of. *Why not?* So I hopped on a plane to the Antigua. Henry picked me up at the airport, chatting all the way to the boat. He was telling me about the communications down there and asked me what my VHF handle (call sign) was.

I told him I had been using "Fallen Angel." Henry started laughing and said that couldn't be any more appropriate. That started *me* laughing. But that's how people knew me, and I did a good job of living up to my name.

Falmouth Harbour, where the boat was anchored, was full of sailboats and big yachts. Very much a yachting community, with people working on charter boats and private boats. It was a very European culture: lots of English, Irish, South African, Australians, and New Zealanders, also known as "Kiwis." I'd never been around that much diversity in people, and I found it to be a lot of fun.

Everybody also seemed to be extremely good-looking, very nice, and sociable. I got to know that little community and found out which people went to which happy hours. Monday, you went to this one. Tuesday, you went to that one.

One day Henry and I turned up at about four o'clock in the afternoon to one of these happy hours. There were tons of people and loud music, with people dancing inside and outside. That bar was popping! It was two-for-one everything. That was THE hangout. If you were anybody, you were there.

So I was having a drink, and I looked out on the dance floor and I spotted a guy. He was about six-foot-one, maybe. Blonde hair, real pretty blue eyes and dimples, and kind of built—not like gym-rat built, but just built. I was just watching him and I thought, *Wow, he's really good-looking.* Henry saw me staring at the guy and started teasing me.

"Oh, you like that guy, the guy who's dancing? I'm gonna go find out who he is," Henry said. I yelled, "Don't you DARE!" Henry would always do embarrassing stuff like that. It was hysterical.

I got talking to some other people, and I noticed that Henry had disappeared. The next thing I knew, I saw him talking to Mr. Blondie. And the next thing I knew after that, Mr. Blondie came up to me and asked me if I wanted to dance. *Oh, my God.*

"Of course," I said, with complete fake confidence. We started dancing to this really loud music. I couldn't hear anything he said. The song ended and I could finally understand him.

"My name's Mark," he said. It sounded like he said "Mock," because he was from England. "I'm Heather," I said. *Ooh, I have always loved me a nice British accent!* It was like a trap door opened and sucked me right in. *Uh-oh, here we go!!*

We danced and danced, drinking and just getting a great buzz on. We walked back to the harbor along this old dirt road. He grabbed my hand and we were walking along, holding hands. I was thinking, *Hmmm, this is different.* He kissed me and I was like, *Wow, this is really different, and I have to say, pretty awesome.*

We got to the harbor he said, "I'll see you tomorrow. Where are you staying?" I told him I was on Henry's boat and he could reach me on the VHF by calling "Fallen Angel."

I suggested we meet for happy hour again—it had gone pretty well the first time—and so we starting hanging out. After the third night of this drinking-dancing-kissing stuff, Mark said he wanted to get away from all the people and go to his boat. It was really late at night, and we boarded the boat and crawled into his bunk bed. You know, one thing led to another, and we eventually fell asleep. It seemed like just a few minutes after that and we both woke up to a noise.

Oh, my God. Someone else is in this bunk bed. Mark laughed and said it was just one of the crew, and we went back to sleep. That was kind of weird, but I think I was half-still-drunk and half-asleep, so I didn't really care.

I snuck out early the next morning thinking that I really liked this guy a lot. I told Henry I thought I was going to marry this guy. That's me... three dates in!

Mark and I started seeing each other very regularly; it was easy and fun and good. After a couple of months, he told me his mom was coming to visit. He was very nervous about it because she was coming for a whole week and he didn't know what he was going to do with her because he had to work. He was honestly kind of a basket case about it.

Mark asked me to help him out, and of course, I agreed. Then he told me, "She doesn't really like Americans." That made me wonder if he had ever mentioned me to her.

"Does she even know about me?" I asked, already knowing the answer. "No, not yet," he said. Then he dropped it on me that she was coming from England and she'd be there *the next day*.

Meanwhile, there had been some talk about a big party up at a fancy hilltop house that everybody was going to. Mark and I had planned to go, but now his mom was coming and he didn't feel he should leave her alone. Seeing that I never turned down a good party, I still planned on going.

Mark was like, "Please don't go. Let me get my mom settled." Well, that was disappointing because I really had my heart set on it. I really, really did. I told Mark he needed to spend time with his mom and that I'd see him after the party. He was not happy.

I went and it was amazing. It turned out that I already knew a few people who were there, but there were tons of people I didn't know. I found out later that it was the vacation home of a mega-famous guitar god. There were women running around topless (including me), even naked people in the pool. We were all just wasted, having a great time.

It wasn't quite as bad as "Girls Gone Wild," but it was pretty damn close. Next thing you know. Mark walked into the pool area. He was asking everyone, "Where's Heather"? *And he had his mom with him.*

He saw me in the pool and called to me. I turned around, not a stitch of clothes on. I looked up and there was Mark and his mom. He was looking at me, dumbfounded. She was glaring at me. He was mouthing, "What the fuck?" Obviously, I couldn't get out of the pool so I said I would catch up with them later. *Oh, my God.*

I don't know when—or how—I got home, but it was very, very late. Mark was so pissed at me the next day, but he was at least polite enough to formally introduce me to his mom.

"Heather, this is my mom, Catherine." I bowed my head in shame and gave her my best, "Nice to meet you!" *Oh, my God.* She was just looking me up and down like I was a "fat slag," a British term, and not a complimentary one. *You are not good for my son.* That was plainly written all over her face.

There was a restaurant at the marina that served a traditional English breakfast: roasted tomatoes, sausage, blood pudding, eggs, potatoes. Heavy-duty food. And that's exactly what I needed because I was so hung over. Mark, Catherine, and I went over there, and were trying to make conversation. It was so uncomfortable, but we got through it, and Catherine left after a few more days. I think I won her over a bit just before she left; I'm not sure. It was maybe a 6 out of 10 in the end.

I have to say I was very relieved after she left. Mark and I went out to happy hour and danced and got shitfaced and everything was back to normal. The next Sunday, we met Mark's friends (who were South African, English, and Irish) at this little bar where they do a nice brunch. That was right around the time when the band Milli Vanilli got caught lip-syncing at all their concerts and everyone found out that they were fakes.

Around one o'clock, we had eaten but were still drinking and everybody was feeling pretty happy. I put my drink down, looked up, and the two Milli Vanilli guys walked in. *Was that them??* So we were drunk, and we all broke into, "Girl, You Know It's True" and everyone turned around to look. You could see that the Vanilli guys were a little embarrassed, but the crowd started clapping, and we were like, "What are y'all waiting for? Sing us a song!"

We knew they didn't really know how to sing. We were just a bunch of yachties at brunch, getting drunk, being obnoxious to Milli Vanilli.

Life in the West Indies was fantastic. Everyone had Sundays off if they weren't working a charter. Sometimes we would do some sailboat racing, which I didn't know how to do but wanted to learn. We'd come back from a day of pleasure sailing and go to the beach and watch the sunset. Some people would say it was a perfect life.

At some point, I couldn't stay on Henry's boat anymore because the owner was coming in. At one of the happy hours I had met this guy, Captain Sean. Tall, lanky fellow with a ponytail. He had an extra berth on his boat, which he nicely offered to me in exchange for maintenance work. His boat was over on the other side of the harbor where some of the bigger motor yachts would dock.

My days consisted of varnishing or waxing, making just enough money for groceries (*aka* wine). I would get a bottle of Beaujolais, a wedge of Brie cheese and a baguette, put it all in my backpack with something to read, and I would head to the beach. Very fancy, you know, just like the Europeans would do it.

Afterward, I'd come back to the boat and put my leftover Brie in the fridge. I did that a few days in a row. I wasn't thinking about how this cheese was getting hot and cold and hot and cold. Well, the next afternoon, I was so sick, I couldn't stop vomiting. Diarrhea, the whole thing, really bad. I realized I had food poisoning, and one of the worst places to have food poisoning is on a 25-foot sailboat where everybody can hear everything that's going on. I was a lot more careful with the cheese after that!

· 35 ·

HITTING THE SLOPES WITH YOU-KNOW-WHO

The West Indies turned out to be a great adventure. Mark and I were a real "couple." I was 31 and he was 21, but he was light years more mature than me!

He introduced me to a lot of his friends, most of whom worked on sailboats. Man, they knew how to party! One couple, Gigi and Ciro, worked on a swanky Perini Navi sailboat, top of the line. Gigi and I hit it off immediately. She was very exotic... Brazilian, I think. Her husband, Ciro, was Italian. Their mate was a Kiwi, from the New Zealand Māori tribe. He lived life on the edge!

These people always seemed to have cocaine, and they became my source. I had a "nose" for where to find it, which led me right to Gigi and Ciro. Mark didn't do any drugs, so I didn't do them in front of him. Gigi would drink wine, or we would drink *caipirinhas*, the national drink of Brazil. Two will knock you on your ass, so I usually had four.

I was comfortable with those people, and we had a fun little family kind of thing. They knew everyone on the island. Gigi and Ciro were well-known and well-liked, and people respected them, kind of like they were the unofficial mayor and mayoress (is that a thing?) of the place.

I remember being invited to go with them to a party at somebody's house after happy hour one night. Some kind of cookout. There were people playing music, and everyone was dressed all bright and chic. It was all very swanky.

As always, parties get into the swing, and the cocaine comes out—but not normally on silver platters, mind you. After a while, things started to wind down and Gigi was talking about going to "Billy's," which happened to be an illegal after-hours bar that was very exclusive. I wanted to go, too. "You're with us," they said, meaning that was how I could get in. *Cool!*

I'd had a couple of "bumps" and a lot of drinks by the time we rolled up to what looked more like a two-story house than a bar. It was nice. There was a pool table, a kind of lounge area, and a bar with only a couple of people there. We got some drinks and I wandered over to the pool table.

I asked Gigi if she wanted to play and said we could ask the other couple of people who were there if they wanted to join us. One of the guys looked pretty wasted.

Gigi whispered, "Do you know who that is? That's (one of the most famous musicians on Planet Earth)! You know, the bloke from (one of the most famous bands on Planet Earth)!"

Oh, that's fucking magic!! I thought. I watched him go down some stairs, and me, after a bunch of bumps and drinks, took the opportunity to go after him. I wanted to meet him. *The nerve I had!!*

As I reached the bottom of the stairs, I saw him go into the loo (bathroom). He pulled something out of his pocket and started putting out a couple lines of blow. He turned around and saw me.

"Hi!!" I said. He gave me a big ol' crooked smile. He looked at the blow and looked at me again. I asked him, "Well, are you going to share?" He just nodded his head and waved me in. I did my bump, and so as not to crowd him (ha!), I went upstairs to look for Gigi. I saw that they were leaving and all I could say was, "Gigi, I just did blow with _____!!"

And so we headed off to our respective boats. Just another fabulous day in Antigua!

· 36 ·

THE RULES OF ENGAGEMENT

Doing coke with a legendary rock star was a hard act to follow, but I had jet-setting of my own to do. HA!

From the West Indies back to the Virgin Islands, Land of Romance for me. Mark and I were happily there at the same time: he was on a sailboat on the west side of one of the islands, and I was on the 108-foot *Whisperwings*, moored on the east side.

It had been a busy day for both of us in preparation for the next trip, and we needed to relax. We met for drinks and dinner on the "his side," which is the more touristy, busy end of the island. The humidity was lower than usual, which made it just perfect for taking an early evening stroll past all the pretty shops. We came up on a jewelry store and wandered inside. It just seemed like the thing to do.

We were just looking around and Mark said, "Heather, if you were to get a ring, what kind would you like?"

That wasn't a total surprise because we had talked about marriage off and on, now and then. We had been together for almost two years. *But a ring? Really?*

The first thing I thought of was my cousin's ring: it was a teardrop emerald with three diamond baguettes on each side. It was stunning! I tried to describe it to Mark, and it became our mission to find one just like it. We went in and out of jewelry stores, window-shopping and dreaming. I didn't see a ring that suited me that day, but I was happy anyway, just because Mark and I were together. That is such a nice memory.

There was never any pressure for either one of us to get married. We kind of knew we would do it eventually, have kids, the whole thing—but we were having too much fun making money and living the nautical life. The downside was that right then, we weren't on the same boat.

My boat was leaving for another island the next day, and Mark was eventually heading to the West Indies. That was going to be a long stint between seeing each other.

Whisperwings' owners, a nice family from Kansas, flew in with their priest, who was a bit of a booze-bag. He could polish off a bottle of Crown Royal in a single night! We anchored in the harbor after a little afternoon cruise, so I still had time to go ashore before dark and hit some of the specialty stores. That night I made dinner for six, starting with Sevruga caviar, followed by some fresh greens and a citrus vinaigrette. The main course was Beef Wellington with Dauphine potatoes and some seasonal vegetables. Dessert was a chocolate pâté with raspberry coulis and whipped cream. Yum!

Here's the dessert recipe. Don't say I never gave you anything, ha!

CHOCOLATE PÂTÉ WITH RASPBERRY COULIS

Ingredients for the Chocolate Pâté:
1 cup salted butter (2 sticks)
3 cups good-quality semisweet chocolate chips
1 tsp. instant coffee granules
1/2 cup granulated sugar
2 large eggs
1 tsp. vanilla extract
1-1/2 cups whipping cream

Line a 9x5 loaf pan with plastic wrap. Melt butter in a large saucepan over hot water or on low heat. Add chocolate chips and coffee granules, stirring constantly until smooth. DO NOT OVERHEAT. Pour into a large mixing bowl. Add sugar and beat until sugar is dissolved. Beat in eggs, one at a time, then mix in the vanilla extract. In a small, chilled bowl, beat whipping cream in until stiff, and gently fold it into chocolate mixture. Turn into the loaf pan. Cover and chill for at least 8 hours or overnight.

Ingredients for the Raspberry Coulis:
Coulis is basically a sauce, but it sounds more fucking fancy to say coulis (coo-lee).

15 oz. frozen raspberries in syrup, thawed
2 T. granulated sugar
4 tsp. cornstarch

Strain berries/syrup through a sieve to remove seeds. In a small saucepan, combine strained berries, syrup, sugar, and cornstarch and heat, stirring constantly, until mixture boils and thickens. Cool and refrigerate. Makes 1-1/4 cups.

To serve: Pour sauce on a plate, top with a slice of pate and finish with a dollop of whipped cream. Serves 8-10.

I was finishing up the dishes and the captain walked in to tell me to look out the port side door. I didn't hear the "port side" part and opened the door that was just off my galley. I looked around, saw nothing, and went back to my business. What impressed me was what a beautiful night it was.

A few minutes later, I heard the captain yelling to me from the wheelhouse. "Heather! Check the port side!" I yelled back that I already had, and he yelled, "No, YOUR left!"

I started giggling to myself, *You goofball, are you ever going to learn which side is port?!* So I went over the actual port side door and opened it to hear, "Hey, beautiful!"

I looked down and there was Mark, in a dinghy. He had his nice shirt on, one of my faves because it brought out the crystal blue in his eyes. One hand was steadying himself on the boat, and the other hand held a bouquet of very pretty roses. *But wait... isn't he supposed to be on his way to the West Indies?* I was confused.

"Hey!!! What are you doing here?" I asked, more excited than confused at that moment. He told me to get in the dinghy, but I couldn't climb over the rail, so I told him to go around to the stern. I was so excited, happy, but also worried because there were guests on the boat. I didn't want to get in trouble. *What the fuck is happening here?*

I asked the captain for permission to go talk to Mark and he was fine with it. I ran through the salon where all the guests were, sitting and enjoying their after-dinner drinks and coffee. It was like something out of a sitcom.

I got to the aft deck and jumped in the dinghy, and we started rowing away from the yacht. Mark looked like the cat that ate the canary. A whole flock of them.

"Let's open some Champagne," he said, just smiling this wicked little smile. I couldn't stop hugging him, I was so glad to see him. He uncorked the Veuve Cliquot. POP!!! "I love you so much, and you look so nice," I said. "But why aren't you on your way to the West Indies?" He told me to wait a minute.

He nervously handed me a glass of that wonderful Champagne, looking so full of love, and near tears. In that little unsteady dinghy, he got down on one knee.

"Heather, I couldn't leave without seeing you, so I bribed your captain to let me come and do this." As he said that, I looked up and there was a shooting star floating across the sky. I looked back at Mark and saw that he was holding a little box, and I was like, *Oh, my God, what is happening right now?*

He said, "Heather, I love you so much and I want to marry you. Will you marry me, please?" He was crying, I was crying, and I threw my arms around him and started kissing him. He asked me if that was a "yes!" I nodded and opened the box, and there was my teardrop emerald ring. I couldn't believe it. It was like an out-of-body experience.

Meanwhile, the guests were up on deck watching this whole thing. The captain had been in on it the whole time. He shined a flashlight on us and I shouted, "I just got engaged!!!" There were hoots and hollers all around, and we both came back up on the yacht.

The owner wanted to make a big party out of it, but Mark was sad to say that he had to leave for the West Indies. *Ugh,* that hurt, but I asked him to stay just for a little bit, out of respect to the owner.

He was a good sport and stuck around for a while. The captain poured the Champagne, and I was busy showing everyone my beautiful ring. I still couldn't believe my eyes. The owner lifted his glass and proposed a toast to us, and then he asked everyone to say what they thought love was. I knew that would make Mark uncomfortable, because he was really shy and hated being put on the spot, but it turned out to be a beautiful thing, with all the ways people described it. Mark and I each said how we loved each other and it was just so romantic. It was a simply unforgettable night.

I just wanted to be alone with Mark. I wanted to consummate that engagement—but as much as I wanted to, I knew he really did have to go. He said his goodbyes, and everyone hugged him... my hug was the longest.

He took off in his dinghy, and I stood there and watched until he was a little dot that finally disappeared over the horizon. I was so in love with that man! The sound of the mechanical winch pulling up his sailboat's anchor carried across the water, and I saw his boat pull out. I watched it sail off until I could no longer see the mast light.

Be safe, Mark, I love you.

· 37 ·

S/V Rocky: Daddy Issues

Thank God, it was a short trip for Mark, and before we knew it, we were together again on another boat in Florida, getting ready for a big adventure. It was a 70-foot sailboat, *S/V Rocky*, which was run by Captain Dane. The three of us were going to take the owner and his family to St. Thomas, and then on to Spain, France, and Greece. Wow!

I had never been to Europe, so I was very excited. Barry DeKalb, the husband, was a very conservative Texas businessman who had sold a bunch of the stores he owned, which landed him a lot of money. Also, as it turned out, it was a very dysfunctional family. There were two kids: an older son and a daughter who was just a boozer and a train wreck. And I thought *I* was bad, HA! I had nothing on that girl.

The daughter was a bit of a self-absorbed socialite, and she really took the cake. Mom was a throwback hippie who would wake up in the morning, take some pills to get out of bed, smoke pot all day, then take pills to go to sleep. I remember this big mop of curly hair she had that was out of control. The son just kind of showed up from time to time but didn't make the entire trip with the rest of the bunch.

Well, the weirdest thing was that the ditzy daughter had a crush on her *father*. I think they call that the "Oedipus complex" or something. I didn't realize it until we were actually in Spain. I noticed that whenever the daughter and the mom were on board at the same time that they would always be fighting. *Always* fighting. Barry was always the one who tried to put out the fires by trying to be nice to both of them.

Things got to the point where the mom and the daughter couldn't even be on the boat at the same time. One night the mom went off the boat after one of their tiffs, so it was just Barry and his daughter, who was already half-wasted on one of her binges.

It was just so weird. He was like 60-ish, and she was around 25. She was rubbing up against her dad, putting her arms around him, hanging all over him. It was very uncomfortable for me to watch. And Barry was clueless. He thought she was just being affectionate.

Well, the drunker she got, the more like lovey-dovey she got. One night she came into the living area wearing her mother's nightgown, and I thought, *That's pretty odd*. I was up kind of late that night and saw her go into her father's bedroom. And I was like, *Holy shit, please don't let that happen*. I didn't think Barry would let that happen. *Did he let that happen?*

The next night, the daughter went out to some club (probably because Daddy turned her down). She was thrown out of the club and got arrested. We were woken up by a phone call at three o'clock in the morning to come and bail her out. Barry went to the police station, and she was all pilled up. She was a drug addict, an alcoholic, a spoiled little rich girl. Not a happy scenario.

I once overheard talk between the mom and daughter that the older son was gay, and that Barry was a bit of a homophobe. They didn't want to tell Barry that his son had a boyfriend; they actually kept it from him, which I thought that was really sad. But that was none of my business. There was just a lot of deep-shit psychological drama on that boat and it affected all of us.

The son decided to join one of the trips, and planned to surprise his dad by bringing his boyfriend. If it had been me, I probably would have done it a little different because we were all on this 70-foot boat, stuck with each other, with nowhere to go.

The son flew over first and had a couple of days alone with this dad. He told Barry he was gay, and I saw Barry start to cry. This was his only son, his pride and joy, and he didn't want his son to be gay. He wanted his son to produce an heir, or whatever. I, for one, would have liked to see this family line come to a dead stop.

After a day or so of getting used to this news, the shock still was there but had worn off a little bit. The son figured that was a good time to spring it on Barry that his boyfriend was coming the next day and they could all spend time together. *Holy shit.* How uncomfortable was *that*? To my surprise, it worked out pretty well, though. Maybe Barry was just in denial. You just never know about people.

· 38 ·

S/V ROCKY: KNEE-DEEP

We left Spain and went on to France, then the Greek Islands. The conditions were really, really windy and the docking situation was tricky coming into Athens. We usually went stern in, too, which added another layer of difficulty. It was just getting dark as we were backing into the dock, and the boat was bouncing up and down on the waves. My job was to get the stern line on, which is the back in the boat. I'd usually time it to jump off the boat, get the line on and clear the dock.

Well, it was really dodgy. I leapt to the dock but the boat lurched way up while I was on the way down, so I fell about ten feet, landing on my knee. I was still trying to get the line on and everyone was shouting, "Heather, get the line on. Get the line on!" I couldn't move my leg, so I pulled myself along, like crawling, and got the line on. The others finally saw that I couldn't get up, so they got the other line on and hoisted me back up onto the boat.

I just bruised it, I thought. Well, of course, the next day my knee was swollen, swollen, swollen and a doctor needed to look at it. Finding a clinic was not easy, and you know, the Greek language is really hard. I learned enough to grocery-shop a little bit but not quite enough to find a medical clinic. I finally got an appointment and got to the clinic (using an umbrella for a crutch), and I waited. And waited. They told me the doctor couldn't see me for hours, so I just left and lived with it.

The next stop was a hilly little Greek island, so hilly that you either had to hike or ride a donkey to get up to the main town. So I found a cane and we took the donkey up. It was such a beautiful island, but it was very physically painful trip for me.

Barry told me his Texas doctor had a doctor-friend in Athens and that when we got back to Athens, he could take a look at my knee. Barry also offered me the chance to go back to Texas with the family and see the top orthopedic surgeon in the country.

Well, at that point, I really didn't want to be around this family anymore. They had put us through the ringer. So when we returned to Athens, I decided to see the Greek doctor. Mark went with me.

The doctor came in and started speaking broken English. I didn't understand much, but I did understand that I apparently blew my knee out and needed surgery. They could do it in Athens and I'd spend two to three days in the hospital. The recovery time would probably be two weeks, all off my feet. *Oh, my God. Do I get operated on in a foreign country?*

There was also that alternative of going back to Texas with the DeKalbs. That made Athens sound pretty damn good.

In the end, I decided I should probably go to Texas, do it right, and just suck it up. So I flew to Texas and stayed at the DeKalb's house. Their butler (this awesome gay guy who was either the houseboy, mom's drug dealer, or both) just couldn't have been nicer. Their house was like eight bedrooms, just huge. Mom collected miniature animals: pigs, llamas, ponies, dogs, you name it. They were *everywhere*. (I can't make this up. I really can't.)

The surgery lasted an hour and then I was supposed to recoup at the DeKalb house for four days. It so happens that Mrs. DeKalb's 50th birthday party had been scheduled during my recuperation period. Barry had hired Michael Bolton and Kenny G to play in their backyard for this big soirée. Pretty schmancy.

I remember waking up the next day, being in so much pain and wishing Mark was there with me. I called him and begged him to come to Texas, and he flew over just in time for the party. For some reason, half the local police department was there as guests. Kenny G and the Cops. The whole thing was extremely surreal.

· 39 ·

S/V Rocky: Disengagement

After a week or so, when I could travel, I went back to Florida and Mark flew back to his boat in Athens to work.

When Mark wasn't around, I'd hang out with our friends just to have the company—nothing hinky, just for companionship. Jamie, this guy I had met in Florida a while back, didn't care that I had a fiancé; he just kept asking me out. He was kind of attractive, French-Canadian—but what turned me off was that he always had hair coming out of the back of his neck. *Gross.* Anyway, he was really insistent about going out, so I finally went out with him. *Mark was in Greece, and I'm going back soon. No harm, no foul,* I thought.

Jamie and I just went out to dinner a couple of times. I thought nothing of it... but maybe I did because I was kind of starting to feel a little attracted to him. I was committed to Mark and still was very much in love with him, but things seemed to be changing a little bit between us. Could have been my drinking, could have been my drugging. Did I have a problem? Yep, but I was still functioning pretty well. I wasn't drinking in the morning to start my day (yet) and getting trashed was still my greatest form of fun. Hindsight's 20/20, you know.

By then, my knee was healed up enough to go back to Athens and *S/V Rocky,* but I wanted to stay in touch with Jamie. In those days everybody stayed in contact by faxing (!), so I got his number told him I would fax him when I got to Greece so we could keep up our "friendship."

None of that changed the fact that I was excited to see Mark; I couldn't wait to see him, but this little buzzy gnat in my head was telling me that something was going on.

Mark picked me up at the airport, and I was shitfaced because I drank so much on the plane. You know, from Miami to Athens is a very long flight. He barely kissed me.

I looked at him like, "What?" and he said, "God, you're wasted and you're gross." Fine, so we drove back to the boat in silence and I just went to bed. I think I woke up the next day asking where Mark was because he wasn't on the boat. I finally saw him and said, "Hey, honey, how are you?"

"Fine," he said as he walked right past me. His coolness was not lost on me.

This was getting to be February, and my birthday was coming up. I was excited, wondering what Mark was going to get me for my birthday and what we were going to do. There was just this nagging bad feeling. He was distant. We had always held hands; we always had a great friendship as well as a great love life and sense of adventure. I really thought he was going to be the one that I was going to marry.

That morning, I remember walking into town with him and he was barely holding my hand.

"Mark, what's going on with you?" I asked, not sure I really wanted an answer.

"Well, you know, I love you, but I'm not in love with you anymore." *What? What? What?*

"I don't know. I feel like we're growing apart," he said. He wouldn't even look at me. I was thinking, *What did I do? What can I do?* I was in fight-or-flight mode. I asked him to tell me what he was talking about, but he just dodged it. I could not get him to talk to me.

After about a month of begging, I threw in the towel. We decided it was probably best for both of us if I left after the last leg of the trip.

Turned out that he had met "some people" in Greece while I was nursing my knee in Texas. I found out much later that "some people" was "some girl."

The second-to-last leg of the trip was to Israel, an epic sail through the Strait of Messina, arriving in the dark.

Israel is probably one of the awesomest places I've ever been, which helped ease the tension of being around this weird family again. At least one cool thing about them was that whenever we got to a new country, they would hire a driver and a car so they could get a local feel for wherever they were. They would always take us with them and we got to see everything they saw for nearly two years, all over the Mediterranean. I got to surf Tel Aviv! The clubbing was amazing. What a wonderful place!

It was finally time to take the boat back to the States, the dreaded "last leg." Mark dropped me off at the airport and we were both crying and crying because we had been together nearly five years, and we were breaking up. He was going off to Acapulco to work on another boat.

"I love you," I said, crying. "I love you, too," he said, crying maybe worse than me. We started to walk away from each other and I turned around like in the movies and said, "Wait for me!!" He just said, "You'll be fine," and he turned away and walked until I couldn't see him anymore.

I found myself standing in the ticket line, feeling just so empty, and out of nowhere this very professional lady came up to me. She looked like some kind of police. Without a word, she pulled me out of the line. *What is up with this?*

"I need to check your bags," she said. I protested, telling her my flight was boarding soon.

Again, she said, "I need to check your bags." Well, this is everything I own—two huge bags that took forever to pack. *Ugh.* She had somebody check my bags and then ordered me to come behind the curtain. I asked why and she explained that they needed to strip-search me. *Wait. You need to WHAT?*

I was already upset because I had just lost my fiancé, and now they were going to strip me, have me bend over and cough, you know, check me for drugs. They wouldn't find any, because I didn't drug when I was on a boat. It was so humiliating and made me so angry. *Another worst day ever!*

Then I saw all my clothes pulled out of my bags and they were announcing over the PA that my flight was boarding. A lady helped me shove everything back in the bags while I was thinking about how ridiculous this all was.

Where's my passport? I need my passport. I asked Police Lady, "May I please have my passport?" I always knew to be nice to these people and treat them with respect, because the minute you didn't, nothing was going to go your way.

So Police Lady handed me the passport along with a promotional airlines pen and said, "Here's a little parting gift for you. So sorry for your inconvenience." I was fucking livid. Fucking *livid*.

After a kind of turbulent flight, Jamie picked me up at the Miami airport. Little did I know that he would turn out to be one of the loves of my life. *Fuck me!*

· 4 0 ·

FINISH LINE: NOT UNTIL THE FAT LADY SINGS

Probably the funniest yachting story is from when I was on this 112-foot motor yacht called *Finish Line*. The captain's name was Kent (crazy, and funny as fuck!). He and I were like Tom and Jerry. No, wait... more like Batman and Robin. It made me forget about Mark, who I heard had got on some 60-foot boat in Mexico.

Nursing a heartbreak was a job in itself. I really thought Mark was going to be the one I married and spent the rest of my life with. So what does somebody who's sad and nursing a heartbreak do? *Drink.*

Finish Line's owner was from Puerto Rico, and he decided he wanted to take the boat over to South America, where he could sport-fish. You have to go through the Panama Canal to get there, so that's what we did: me, Captain Kent, the owner, the mate, and the stewardess.

Captain Kent and I fell right into the local scene, just like we'd never met a stranger. We were just tearing up Puerto Rico. My best friend Amy came from Virginia Beach to visit me for a week and we rented a car, driving all around the island.

We stayed in the local *paradores*, little guest houses that were very inexpensive. One night we went out to a Japanese place for dinner and drank sake until we got raging drunk. Oh, my God, it was so much fun, and it let me forget Mark for a while.

I still wanted the relationship to work, and so I kept calling him, using the old international phone cards that people used to use for long-distance. I was kind of spinning out of control trying to re-glue this relationship back together from 2,000 miles away. I probably called him too much, but he didn't seem to mind.

"Mark," I said, with maybe a little desperation in there, "I need to see you." This was about two months after we had our teary goodbyes at the airport.

He was like, "Yeah, but I gotta work." I insisted that we needed to see each other, don't you know? I was grasping at straws. So I just announced that I was flying to Acapulco for a few days. And I did. I think Kent could see that I was hurting and needed to get away, so he gave me his blessing.

I was scheduled to fly into Mexico City and stay three days. Well, they canceled my flight, and the next one wasn't until the following day, chopping a whole day out of my time with Mark. I was all broken up, calling him and crying about it. We had the best phone sex ever on that call!

After what seemed like the longest flight ever, I called Mark from the Mexico City airport and he gave me directions to the marina where he worked. Of course, all the locals spoke Spanish, but I did not. I showed up at the marina office and waited, waited, waited.... waited, waited some more. I saw his boat come in and I was so nervous. I just wanted to run down the dock and kiss him and hug him.

He wasn't coming up to the office. He knew I was there. *What was going on with that?* I thought, *Well, I'll just walk down there,* not absorbing how rude he was actually being to me.

I walked up and I was like, "Mark!" He just kind of looked at me and said, "Hey."

Hey? We used to hold hands and kiss everywhere in public; we didn't care. Now he could barely give me a hug. Red flags started popping up all over the place. *Was he leading me on again?*

He asked, "What are you doing here? I got to clean the boat. Here's the address for the house and some money for a cab. Go on and I'll meet you there."

The look on my face must have been like one of those sad-puppy looks on a viral video. *Why didn't he want to see me?*

Didn't matter, I did what he said. I went up to his house and dropped my bag in his room. I looked around and something was so off. There were no photos of us—of me—anywhere. I started looking around for them, because that used to be a big deal for us, taking photos and putting them out. We had tons of pictures of the two of us, so where the hell were they? I was about to stop snooping when I saw a shoebox on his closet shelf. I got it down, and there were the photos, hundreds of photos. I spread them all over his room, because I'm that girl.

I waited another four hours for him to come home. I was all by myself in this condo, waiting and waiting, looking at the photos. I changed my clothes and changed them again, trying on every sexy pose possible. Finally, I just put my bikini on.

Mark eventually made it home and I asked him why there weren't any pictures of us out.

"I don't spend that much time here," was the lame answer, along with some other excuses. This did not feel good.

We went down to the pool, had a drink or two, and started making love in the pool. It was just amazing, like we really reconnected. We decided to go out and get some dinner and some more drinks, so we went upstairs to change. I got in the shower and he went the other way, down the hall.

I shouted above the noise of the water. "Aren't you gonna come join me?" I heard him start walking away. "I've got to make a phone call," he said. I was thinking that this was really feeling odd after just feeling so great.

At the restaurant, Mark told me his job was pretty demanding and he was tired. I kept asking him if he was OK, and if we were OK. I think I asked if we were OK three or four times. He was like, yeah, yeah, yeah, we're OK. Well, it wasn't very comforting.

He changed the subject and said he would show me around the town the next day. At that point I was too tired to push it any further. We went back to his house, went to bed, and made love again. Everything felt so unsettled and I felt like a yo-yo on a string.

At six o'clock in the morning the phone rang. "Got to go to work," he said.

"Well, did you tell your boss that your girlfriend was here? Maybe I could come on the boat and spend some time with you there?" All I heard was a mumble about the boss not liking visitors on the boat.

Well, I'm Heather, so I kept at it. "Can't you tell him that I'm only in town for one more day?" Even I could hear how needy I sounded, but I wouldn't let it go.

"Not really," he said. It was crushing. *So this is our relationship now?* Mark suggested I go watch the cliff divers and wander around town and said he'd be back later that night. Very nonchalant. *Are you kidding me?*

"I gotta do what I gotta do," he said, just blank, no emotion. In that moment, I knew that we had lost whatever it was that we had, but I wanted to salvage it. I spent the whole day obsessing about it.

Mark walked in the door around dinnertime without a care in the world. We were supposed to go to dinner on my last night there. I had a taxi coming to get me at five in the morning so we made it an early night.

It was all so awkward. We went to dinner, we went to bed, the taxi came. Just like that. He walked me out and *kissed me on the cheek*. Not even like a big hug. "OK, then, goodbye." And he walked back to the house. It was like an out-of-body experience.

All the way to the airport I was thinking, *Well, that was fucked up*. I didn't even know what was happening. There was no explanation, no reason, no way to understand his behavior toward me.

Well, to make a long story short, back in Puerto Rico everybody seemed to have the big clue that I did not have, and that was that Mark was cheating on me... again.

It seems he had a Spanish tutor in Mexico, and she apparently taught him what *mamada* meant early on. *Why wouldn't he break things off with me? Why not tell me?* Then I learned it had been going on for a *year.* It took me a very long time to forgive him for that. Just like Andy, another man who devastated my life.

· 4 1 ·

Finish Line: Terrorist for a Day

Finish Line was getting ready to set sail, so I tried to turn my attention to my job, but I was just sad, another chunk of my heart ripped out of my chest. That's when I was really drinking a lot.

After all the Mark ruckus, we finally left Puerto Rico. We got to the first lock, a beautiful freshwater lake called Gatun Lake. You could jump in and the water was so refreshing, especially when you were used to saltwater. After I finished all of my morning chores, Kent and I decided we would go and check out some of the little islands in the lake.

On a quick trip to the hardware store, we discovered some gems called Cuba Libres (amazing rum and Cokes in a little can). We were like, *SCORE!* We bought about eight cases of these little V8-like cans that were about three-quarters rum with a little Coke in them. Kent and I packed the cooler full of those Cuba Libres for our adventure, and off we went.

He spotted a dock, and we pulled in right under the sign that said, "NO TRESPASSING." To me that meant, "Come on in, Kent and Heather!" I had my nice Nikon camera, and we were just walking around, wondering what this place was. Kent said he thought it might have something to do with electricity for the lock (which, of course, would be highly sensitive information).

We hiked all the way up to the high spot on the island so I could take pictures of the view, and of Kent. All of a sudden, we heard, "HEY, what are you guys doing? Get out of there!"

I looked down to see three guys—big guys—with guns pointing at us and yelling really loud. "You're trespassing! Stop what you're doing, NOW!"

Kent and I started to run as fast as we could. It seemed like it took just a few seconds to get back to the dinghy, jump in, and haul ass back to the boat.

The mate and the stewardess were bitching about how long we'd been gone. They kept calling us on the radio because they wanted to go to shore to go running, and they needed the dinghy to get there. When we came speeding up in the dinghy, they thought we were racing back to accommodate their jogging schedule. They had no idea what had happened.

By now, the Feds had a description of the dinghy so when it pulled up to the little island, the officers were waiting for them, guns drawn.

"STOP! Get out and get on your knees!" they yelled at our crewmates, who were clueless. They must have wondered what the hell we had done.

Kent and I were just laughing our asses off when we heard a call come in on the radio. It was the mate.

"Hey, the police are here and they want to know what you guys were doing on that land." I didn't know what to say, so I said, "Tell them we weren't there."

Remember, we had been drinking our little Cuba Libres and just thought the whole thing was hilarious. We were pretty much shitfaced. A Fed got on the line and said they needed to see us, because the mate just told them it was Kent and I who were there earlier.

Mr. Fed said they would be sending the mate out with the police to escort us back to the island. *Fuck, we're gonna be thrown in some Panama jail and we're never gonna get out.*

I was ordered to bring my camera. Well, I didn't want to bring my camera because the pictures were on it, so I took out the film roll, put in a new one, and put the lens cap on, and I took the camera back over to the little island.

We played stupid. I said, "I don't know anything. Yeah, we were there, but we were scared when you guys started shouting at us. We didn't know." I guess they bought it, because we didn't go to jail that day. Crisis averted.

We made the trip to South America, and the owner did his sport-fishing. I made lots of sushi with all the fresh fish we caught. There is nothing like it!

· 42 ·

FINISH LINE: ACCIDENTS WILL HAPPEN

I should note that every yacht has an agent, so if you go out of the country, the agent will help you clear customs and things like that. The agents would always tell us to stuff your passport in your socks or shoe when you leave the boat.

On the way back from South America, we stopped over for the night before going to the Caymans the next day. We left to go to dinner, and I put my passport in my shoe, out of habit. As I lifted my leg over the edge of the boat, my passport fell out of my shoe into the dark water. I yelled, "KENT, KENT! Get a light! Come on! I just dropped my passport!!"

We looked and looked, but the current was running and there was no way. It was like eight o'clock at night. *Fuck, what am I going to do without my passport?* We called the agent, who was extremely pissed off to be bothered at night, but thankfully, he talked to Customs in Panama and convinced them to let me leave. That solved one problem, but how was I going to get entry into the Caymans?

I have a nice, you know, angelic face, so they let me in but said I'd have to get a passport before I could leave the Caymans. "You can't leave without one," they said. OK, so I was wondering how I was supposed to get to Miami to get a passport if I couldn't leave without a passport? *Ack!*

I called the Miami passport authorities and was able to get a rush request through. Somehow it worked and they let me out of the Caymans and back into Miami, where my Danish friend Silja picked me up in her boyfriend's brand-new convertible Mustang.

On the way to Silja's, we decided to stop for a drink and we parked in some random not-parking area. We didn't want to pay for parking, so we just parked somewhere. We went and had a couple of drinks, did a couple lines, and went back to the car.

We came back to the car to see that the whole back window was smashed. *Oh, my God, what the FUCK!* We were scared. I was sure Silja's boyfriend was going to kill me. All the way home, I was doing lines right out in the open as we were driving on the interstate. We got there and made up some big story about what had happened and I am happy to say that her boyfriend did not kill me.

There were many more adventures on *Finish Line*. Captain Kent and I took her all over: through the Caribbean, the Bahamas, and all the way to Mexico.

Like I said, Kent and I liked to drink a lot together. One night we had been drinking after dinner and decided to go to the pool at the marina. I got in, and I kept egging Kent on to get in with me. For some reason, he wouldn't, so I thought I would just pull him in. With a drink in one hand, I jumped up out of the water to grab his foot. My hand slammed into the metal railing around the pool. *Oh, mother FUCK. I just smashed the shit out of my hand.*

We went back to the boat, and the whole way back my hand was just swelling up and swelling up. I had ice on it all night, thinking about how I had to get up and cook in the morning. I could barely move my hand, it was gross black-and-blue. And now I had to tell the boss I couldn't cook. *UGH!*

"Heather, if you weren't drinking, this wouldn't have happened!", he yelled. *What? We were both drinking.* Blaming each other wasn't making it any better, so he took me to the hospital, where the doctor said I had broken my hand. He put a cast on it that went almost all the way up to my fingertips. All I could remember was how I broke the same damn hand when I was little and how it messed up my handwriting. Now it was broken again and was messing up my job.

How the fuck am I supposed to cook? Imagine trying to open a Ziploc bag, or trying to open a jar of something, or trying to hold a spoon. It was really tough because I was right-handed, and of course, I broke my right hand. All I could do was give it my best effort and not complain.

We eventually took the boat back to Florida, and I quit *Finish Line*. Why? I don't know, because *I don't remember*. I have remained friends with Kent, so when I decided to write this book, I asked him if he would tell me about some of the bad stuff I didn't remember.

"Well," he said, "one thing I recall is that the owner came to the boat one afternoon. He kept a case of Absolut vodka on board. He noticed that three bottles were missing, and he was demanding that I tell him where his vodka went. I said I didn't know. I confronted you, and you said you didn't take it."

I didn't drink Absolut, but maybe I did and just didn't remember. Anyway, when Kent tried to bust me for taking the vodka, I apparently quit. Just quit.

Later I recalled that I *did* drink that Absolut to blot out all the sadness over finding out Mark had been cheating on me for a year. It was clear that my alcoholism was getting pretty bad. Even I could see that.

· 43 ·

GOLDMINE, AND CAPTAIN SAM REDUX

Over the next couple of years, I kind of drifted around. Mostly I was on a boat named *Goldmine*. I was still drinking a lot but thought I still had a handle on it. Strangely, for all the pain-in-the-ass the *Goldmine* owners were, I think their micromanagement of just about everything gave me some structure to my life and that helped me be a little more in control of my drinking. That was good for me, made me feel like I had my feet on the ground.

Goldmine was a kosher boat because the owners were Jewish. This was a whole new education in food. I had to learn how to make challah (egg bread) and a Friday night Shabbat (Sabbath) meal. I got pretty good at matzo ball soup! It was doubly difficult because the owners' grandson was allergic to *everything*.

During one dinner prep, I was super-high on Stacker 2s, an energy supplement that made me feel like I'd done a lot of cocaine. Normally, I would drink to calm down, but the owners didn't drink so there was no alcohol in the galley and I didn't do drugs on my boats... but leave it to me to find a substitute. I was bouncing off the walls and was late getting dinner together (a no-no for the Shabbat meal). The wife kept coming to check on me and was making me really paranoid.

That woman drove me nuts, so I spent as much time in the marina as I could. One night I was drunk at some restaurant (not exactly out of character for me) and met this hot guy who was working down in the marina. He came over to me, said something in my ear, and kissed me. He wanted to know if I would go skinny-dipping with him, and of course, I thought it was a great idea to do that with a total stranger. We were about to "get into things," and for some reason I asked him how old he was.

"Sixteen," he said, with a cute smile. Well, I put the brakes on that pretty fast. When we pulled out the next day, the captain said, "Don't worry, Heather. Next time I'll make it a point to dock near a high school!" I guess word travels fast. Too funny!

Goldmine eventually came back into Florida for a break, so I took a freelance gig in New York. We were busy docking the boat after a day trip, and at the same time I stood up to tie a line, I saw the cool racing sailboat I used to work on, *Redux*. Captain Sam was standing on the fore deck and saw me at the same time.

"Heather, my God, how are you??" He seemed honestly happy to see me, and I thought he looked really good. Sam and I never had a big-deal friendship of any kind, but we did have a really good working rapport.

But—there was always kind of *something*, a little chemistry, in spite of the fact that he could be a hard-ass. He was the one, remember, who said work was never finished on a sailboat? So it was interesting when Big Bad Captain Sam very nicely asked me to come over for a party later, which I did after my dinner service was wrapped up.

About the first thing out of his mouth was about how he and his wife Allie weren't doing too well and that he didn't know what to do. I think they had very recently split, from the sound of it. Well, that was as good of a reason as any to get drinking, and we drank just enough to fall into bed together. I think it shocked both of us, but at the same time, we were very, very pleasantly surprised. It was the most amazing sex ever!

Oh, my God, what the hell, a married guy? Sam was just the first of several married men I fooled around with. There was a very predictable pattern of bad judgment taking over when alcohol and drugs were involved. Anyway, Sam and I started this crazy, lust-filled affair. He flew me up to Connecticut once and we had the most amazing weekend... we barely got out of bed.

When we were in a restaurant, we were all on top of each other. Yep, we were that annoying, gross couple who were just sucking face in front of everybody. People were probably thinking, *Get a fucking room.* You're probably thinking the same thing reading this, but that's the way it was. We just had this chemistry and could not get enough of each other. *Man.*

To fuck things up even more, Jamie came back into the picture. He was the Florida guy I was sorta seeing while my ex-fiancé Mark was away. So now I was juggling Sam and Jamie, trying like hell to have some kind of stable relationship but going about it in a really cockeyed way. At least Jamie wasn't married.

My theory is: *When you're in a mess, run!* So I decided to leave *Goldmine* for a new adventure... back in Mexico.

· 4 4 ·

AM I DEAD YET?

Everything was black.

Why do I feel like I've been swimming for forever? I feel wet. It's dark. I don't know where I'm at. I felt rain dripping on my face. *Was it rain?* I struggled to open my eyes, but I couldn't. I didn't know what was happening... *Was I just dreaming?*

Then I felt something on my face. *What was that?* I tried again to open my eyes... *Why was it so hard to do?* My eyes felt glued shut and I couldn't seem to move my arms. I finally opened my eyes in the pitch black, and there was a dog licking my face.

I didn't know why I was all wet. I had been swimming, or something. I didn't know. I needed to get up; I didn't feel very well.

I start to see around me a little bit. I was in a house, and there were dogs, just looking at me. I got up and I could not figure out why I was all wet; my head, my shirt? *Where the hell am I? Am I still in Cozumel?*

Going outside seemed like a good idea, so I walked out and had a little flash. There were four little cottages in front of me, and then I remembered: *I'm in Mexico on a boat job. That cottage is Rico's. He's my friend and he will help me.* I was pretty out of it, not really knowing what I was doing, and I knocked on Rico's door.

The door opened and a man's voice screamed, "OH MY GOD! OH MY GOD, HEATHER! Who did this to you?!"

That was very confusing because I didn't know what he meant. I just said I didn't feel well.

The man, who was indeed Rico, asked me where I had been. I didn't know that, either. He told me he was going to get me a clean shirt. He also said he didn't want me to look in the mirror. He pleaded, "Promise me that you will not look in the mirror!"

I had been wearing one of the mate's shirts, a Versace electric-blue thing, which I had borrowed without his knowledge. I figured he wouldn't miss it because he was in the hospital after rolling the yacht's Jeep. He had blown his collarbone out.

Rico came back with a man's shirt and instructed me to go in the bathroom and change, but not to look in the mirror. Well, when somebody tells you not to, you're probably going to.

I went into the bathroom and took off the shirt. *Should I look? Why would Rico say that?* Maybe I should look, maybe something's wrong. He was *screaming* it, after all.

I looked.

I was covered in blood. My head, my hair, just matted with blood. There was blood on my face, all over the shirt. I screamed and screamed and SCREAMED, about to pass out.

Rico came running, knowing I had looked. He was mad that I had, but he was worried at the same time. He kept asking what had happened and I just kept saying I didn't know.

He tried to clean up my face before we went, but I guess it didn't help much because when we got to the hospital the people there were like, *Oh, my God, what happened?*

The doctor asked if I had lost consciousness and I said I thought so. I didn't know what day it was, or what time it was. In a few minutes they had me on a gurney and were wheeling me in to get X-rayed.

Turns out I fractured my skull. *Hmmm.* I don't know how I could have fractured my skull. They shaved the back of my head and put in a bunch of stitches (the scar looks like the Star of David), and then I was admitted. I kept passing out, probably from all the blood I had lost—who knows how much.

It just so happened that I was in the same hospital as Jimmy, the broken-collarbone mate whose shirt I borrowed. People were coming to visit both of us and everyone kept asking me where I was the night before. I didn't know. I couldn't remember anything. All I could feel was a dull, throbbing pain in my head.

They had me on morphine, and more morphine. I was in heaven! Just push that button, push that button, give me more and more! *But how the hell did I fracture my skull?* It was so strange that I couldn't remember anything.

Then little bits started coming back. I thought I had been at one of the bars, one with live music. I was there with a friend, having some drinks. Another girl I knew and this big German guy came up to us and wanted to buy us a round, so we let them buy us some Heinekens.

I remember saying I needed a ride somewhere, maybe to Randy's house (a guy I was seeing then) and I was in a car with the big German guy. He started groping me and I threw myself out of the passenger's side door. I just opened the door and jumped out and hit my head on a rock.

That's all I could remember. It was all a big mystery.

A couple of friends came up to the hospital and were trying to get me to describe this guy who attacked me. What did he look like? All my friends were looking for this big German guy.

Randy, who had just gotten back from a trip, came right to the hospital because Rico had told him I'd been hurt. He asked the same thing everyone else did, and I gave him the same I-don't-know answer. Randy wanted to know if I had been at his house. He was asking really urgently, but I didn't know why. He kept telling me to think hard and I said it hurt my fucking head to think hard.

"I need to know because there's a big pool of blood at the bottom of my stairs," he insisted. And then it started coming back to me.

Randy lived in an old kind of Spanish style house, made of adobe with those red roof tiles. I had left the bar—by myself, no big German guy—and walked over to Randy's house, you know, for a booty call. I walked up the 16 adobe steps to his room, at the top, yelling, "Randy! Randy!" I opened the door and realized he wasn't there; he was out of town. I shut the door and turned around on my boot heel, which caught the top of the stairs. I tumbled over, and over, and over, hitting my head again and again on the hard stairs, then landing face-up, head-first, at the bottom.

Someone asked the bartenders if they knew what time I had left, and from that we figured out that I was unconscious for about two hours, just bleeding at the bottom of the stairs.

What a crazy thing to happen. While people were running around looking for some German guy to kill, the truth was that I went over to my boyfriend's place and did a dead-drunk-fall down the damn stairs.

I did have a boat job during that mishap, one of my last freelance gigs. The boat belonged to a very rich man who owned a big Mexican beverage company. He loved his tequila. He'd come down in the morning and have a glass of it and just sip it, like how Americans drink OJ.

The captain was a bit of an asshole. He was this Australian guy, very suave and arrogant. He would flirt with me quite a bit, and I thought he was kind of cute in an obnoxious way, but he was just an asshole from Day One. I got my revenge by drinking the tequila when no one was around.

Anyway, Captain Asshole came to my hospital room to find out what happened to his chef, and I told him I fell down some stairs. All he could say was, "Jesus Christ,

Jimmy's in the other room. You're in this room. You know what, you need to get off my boat." He fired me in the hospital room. I couldn't believe it. *Are you always such an asshole, or is today some kind of special occasion?*

What the fuck do I do now? Again, I had no money. I did have a few friends because I had been in Cozumel for about a month. I ended up staying at one of their places because when they released me, I still couldn't do a lot and had to stay pretty still for about four days. You know what they say about houseguests after three days, so I started thinking about where to go. I wasn't really ready to go back to Florida, but that's what I did.

Yep, I got better, but that fall down the stairs was one of the scariest things that ever happened. I don't know what it is with me and Mexico and hospitals, but for sure, the common denominator was alcohol.

· 45 ·

THE BAD PENNY

After landing back in Florida, I decided to just go freelance—pick up a job, go out for a week or two, and not be tied down.

Jamie and I hooked up almost immediately after my return to Florida. He went from zero to full-time boyfriend in about three seconds. Sam became an afterthought. That meant all my co-dependence could be focused on Jamie, who was hot, handsome, and a top dog in the yachting industry.

He took me to all the nice restaurants, you know, and we had great, great sex. He dressed nice, and he worked out, so he looked good in those good clothes. He was a fun guy and loved adventure. It was all very grand and sweet, like a fairy tale.

Jamie did no drugs at all, which should have been good for me, but I still did drugs with my friends. Sometimes he'd come home, and I'd be out; I'd roll in around four o'clock in the morning, my heart racing because I was so coked up. I didn't want him to see that part of me, but it was hard to hide it.

Jamie was both a world-class chef and a yacht builder, and at that time, he was overseeing the construction of a boat in Holland. He was flying back and forth a lot, which meant leaving his car at the airport. I didn't have a car then, so I was always stranded.

"When I get back, I'm going to buy a Jeep and you can keep it at your place so you'll have something to drive while I'm gone," he offered, which I thought was pretty nice.

"Then we can go do some off-road trips." We had talked on and off about going to Disney World, and now we could do it in the new Jeep. Jamie even showed me a picture of it: a green Jeep Cherokee with tan leather interior.

He returned from Holland and we planned the trip all out. Come the day we were going to leave, he showed up in a rental car—not the Jeep.

"Where's the Jeep?" I asked. I was really looking forward to driving it. I got a bunch of sideways answers and never did find out what happened. It seemed strange at the time, and after that, a little part of me always wondered if he was hiding something from me.

Anyway, the two of us drove off in the rental car and went to Disney World, the first time we had ever traveled together. It was a ton of fun. I was really falling for Jamie, but I was still kinda hurt from Mark, I have to say. It took me a very, very long time to say those "three little words" to Jamie.

· 46 ·

MELON MAN

At that same time, many of my European yachtie friends were all back in Florida. They were staying at the local marina, which was not a blessing; it was more of a curse, because they loved to party. It wasn't anything to spend $500 on the weekend. Fridays you'd go out to Bailey's, then Saturday maybe to the steakhouse where all the yachties hung out. Sunday brunch was usually downtown, where you could drink all the Champagne you could handle for fifty bucks. That buzz was always my lead-in to start looking for the drug man. It was an expensive lifestyle.

I finally got my friends to tell me where they were getting their coke so I wouldn't always have to buy it off them, or just always ask them for it. They let me in on their drug man, who was pretty cool. He sold flowers in the street median, at a stoplight. If you told him you wanted two flowers, he'd give you an eight-ball. One flower equaled a gram. You paid him, and he'd put the drugs in a little baggie and hide it in a bouquet.

My backup was the "Melon Man," who was awesome. He had a farm stand; you know, the kind of roadside stand where you get tomatoes and melons. This guy also had cocaine. There, it was an order of "three tomatoes" that got you an eight-ball in a melon. I became that guy's worst nightmare, constantly buying drugs between freelance jobs. I think he was worried that my too-frequent visits were going to tip off the cops.

Once I got there too late and the Melon Man's stand was closed for the day, so I called him and asked him if I could come to his house. He knew me well enough, so he said OK, and I went. He was an old hippie with a really long beard. Nothing attractive about him at all... he was kind of creepy, really. I knocked on the door and I heard, "Who is it?" I said who I was. I was on a mission, just wanted to get my drugs and get home.

He opened the door and he was buck-naked! *Oh, my God,* I'm thinking, *Shit, what am I gonna have to do for these drugs?*

"Just come on in," he said. I pointed out that he was naked, and he said, "Well, I guess I'll put some pants on." And he was just wandering around his house, which was a total mess, looking for his pants. *Man.* He told me to have a seat but I didn't even want to sit on anything in that house. I was so skeeved out... anything to get my drugs and get out of there. He gave me a line and a beer, then he found his pants, in that order.

After about 45 minutes of this, he gave me my drugs and I hauled ass out of there. Those trips became the norm for me. What a girl will do for drugs!

· 4 7 ·

THE LIGHT BULB EXPLODES

I lived a double life for a long time, trying to keep my shit together and also keep Jamie from knowing about my drug habit. But maybe I wasn't the only one with a double life.

After the weird Jeep/no-Jeep incident, we had a few rough patches because sometimes he'd tell me things that didn't add up like they should. He'd tell little lies, like say he would be somewhere when he wasn't, and I'd find out about it. My feeling about that was, look, if you're gonna lie to me, you can't be in my life.

So many times we'd fight, then he'd show up at my house with lots of presents and whatever, and charm his way back into my bed. And in true Heather fashion, I was like, *OK. I'm up for some more emotional abuse because Emotional Abusers 'R' Us.* My mom did the same thing; she went back to my dad countless times, no matter how hard he promised he wouldn't drink anymore.

I was going out and coming back in on a string of freelance charter jobs, partying a lot, and you know, still kind of heartbroken over Mark even though I had Jamie. Then a real awakening came to me. It was on a provisioning trip to a Publix supermarket in the middle of the night for a charter that left at eight o'clock. That morning.

It was a small charter, just four guests. *Piece of cake, right?* I'd talked back and forth with the owners, who were very to the "T" about what they wanted on the provision sheet. I had always prided myself on making everything from scratch, and there I was, staring at the Sara Lee cakes in the freezer case, thinking that I could garnish the hell out of them and pass them off as "homemade."

At that moment, the light bulb didn't just go off; it blew *up.*

What the fuck are you doing, Heather? You're in the grocery store at two o'clock in the morning because you couldn't stop doing drugs long enough to do your job. Your standards have gone down the drain. What the hell, Heather?

That was the first time it really sunk in that I had a problem.

I did the charter, but it was a painful trip. I couldn't drink and I didn't have any drugs for four or five days because I knew I had to do my job. *Jesus,* it was horrible. I found myself chugging the guests' unfinished glasses of wine or liqueur just to get that "warm glow," just to take the edge off.

That was the routine for a while. Take a job, stay reasonably straight for the job, come back and party up a storm. I would be back in Florida on my friend's boat at the marina, still partying and playing loud music at six in the morning, still wearing my clothes from the night before, while other people were getting ready to go to work.

I did the Walk of Shame many, many, many times. I looked for drug dealers in the middle of the night, just to keep the party going. I feel like I didn't eat for like eight years, but I'm sure I did or I wouldn't be here. The scales were tipping and the drugs were now more in control than I was.

· 48 ·

GOOD JAMIE

Meanwhile, Jamie was still going back and forth to Holland because this boat-building project was taking forever. We still fought about stuff because I didn't think he was being straight with me and who knows what he was doing over there. (*That's rich, coming from me!*)

One afternoon he showed up in my yard, where I was just laying out in the sun. A couple of days before that, we had gotten into another argument and I told him never to call me again, to just leave, get out of my life. I don't even remember what the fight was about.

I looked up at him and saw that he had an armful of roses—two dozen white ones.

Those have always been my favorite, along with 'Minuet'.

"Heather, I love you so much," he said. "I don't wanna fight with you anymore. What can I do to make this better? What can I do to get you back in my life?"

We sat there and talked for like forever. He said everything would be different, and of course, he squirmed himself right back into my good graces.

That night we were laying in bed, and he said, "You know what? I've saved up so much money. I know you've been thinking about opening up your own fitness center. Why don't we make our dreams come true? Why don't we get out of the yachting industry and go to Maine?"

Early on in our relationship, Jamie told me he was from Quebec and that his father had a restaurant there. His family also had a big house in Camden, Maine. I guessed that was what he was talking about.

I kind of opened my eyes wide and absorbed the shock of that huge, life-changing question. Being such an active girl, I'd always had a fantasy about having my own fitness center, and I was absolutely thrilled at the thought of making that happen.

After about a half a second I knew at that point in my life I was looking to be rescued. I was looking for a new start, a new place. Lately I had been going down a rabbit hole, and I was thinking, *Oh my God, now I finally have a chance to have my fairy tale. I've got my Prince Charming, my castle, money. Everything I've ever wanted.*

I said, "Jamie, that would be so amazing... can we really do that?" He assured me that we could and suggested that we take a month and plan everything all out. He would pack up his apartment; I would take care of wrapping up our boat jobs. It was going to be so great. Then he said, "Why don't you fly up to Virginia Beach and see your friend Amy for a week or so?"

It was a little odd, but it was a great idea. I hadn't seen Amy for a long time. In the meantime, Jamie said, he would fly to Quebec and in a week he'd meet me there and introduce me to his parents. That was perfect! What a great, great plan! So I packed up my Florida life and put everything in storage except the clothes I was going to take with me.

All the way to the airport, I babbled to Amy about the man of my dreams. She was truly excited for me and said I had never looked so happy. I explained that even though it wasn't a real proposal, I was sure that when we got to Maine, he would have a ring for me and everything, and he would do it properly.

Jamie would call me at Amy's every night and tell me how much he loved me, how he couldn't wait to spend his life with me. Then he would ask me to put Amy on the phone, and he would tell her the same thing. He would go on and on about how he was going to take care of me and give me everything I never had. This was *it*.

· 4 9 ·

BAD JAMIE

That week flew by, and Amy took me to the airport and dropped me off. That was before online check-in and airport kiosks, so I made sure I had the right airline and confirmation number Jamie had given me.

I practically skipped up to the ticket counter, I was so excited to start my new life. "I'm Heather Gaines," I announced. "Here's my driver's license and my flight confirmation number. Can you please check me in?"

The agent clacked on her keyboard and looked at the little terminal screen and declared, "I'm sorry, we don't have that confirmation number, ma'am."

I made sure I was at the right airline ticket counter. "The person who bought my ticket told me this was the airline," I insisted. The agent repeated that she didn't have a reservation under that number and said I should try a different airline.

OK, so I went to *every single airline ticket counter* and no one had my reservation. I started to panic.

This was also still the age of pay phones and calling cards. I called Jamie's dad's house in Quebec. *Ring, ring, ring. Answer the damn phone.*

"Hello?" It seemed like three years later. "Hello, is anyone there?" I was guessing it was Jamie's dad.

"Is Jamie there?" I asked. "Jamie's not here." I tried again in 30 minutes. "Jamie's not here." Again. "Jamie's not here." It was so completely frustrating.

Could I have been at the airport on the wrong day? I retraced my route to all the ticket counters to see if there was a reservation in my name for ANY day.

THERE WAS NO RESERVATION.

After about two hours, it all started to become painfully clear. I couldn't get in touch with Jamie because he didn't want me to get in touch with him. There was no fucking ticket. This was all a sham. That sociopath just fucking ripped my heart out. He promised me the world and then yanked it out from under me. That fucker ruined my life; he stole my joy and killed my soul.

Mother fucker!!! Now I know why they say everyone is capable of killing someone if they're pushed far enough.

I called Amy to come back to the airport to get me, and I was just a crying heap. I didn't know what the fuck to do. I had like a hundred dollars to my name. I had no car, no job, no place to live. *What was I going to do?*

And that, right there, sent me into the biggest, deepest depression I'd ever been in. It was to the point where I was thinking about suicide.

I kept trying to call Jamie, but the motherfucker never called me back. Never fucking heard from him.

Amy and her husband Bill took me in out of sheer pity. I spent my time just drinking all day. They loved wine and always had lots around, but after a week they were sure going to notice that their supply was going way down. That was not going to fly for very long.

I was even taking quarters out of their change jar and hiding wine bottles under my bed so I could drink in my room without them judging me. I always thought everyone was judging me. At that moment, my soul was black. I really didn't think I had anything to live for.

FAST-FORWARD: A PITCHER FOR YOUR THOUGHTS

A year later, my sister and I were sitting at Flannagan's in Fort Lauderdale, enjoying a beer and chatting up the bartender. I looked around the bar and saw something I couldn't possibly have seen. Funny, my eyes must have been playing tricks on me. Was that *Jamie?*

Elizabeth looked at my face and realized something was up. "Heather! What's wrong?" she asked. What she saw was my expression filling up with rage... it was all coming back again, at warp speed.

"It's fucking *Jamie*," I said, under my breath.

"Oh, shit," said Elizabeth, in a voice even quieter than mine. What happened next was just like an out-of-body experience.

Revenge is best served cold, right? I hesitated one second before I asked the bartender to pour me a pitcher of beer. I grabbed the pitcher and made a beeline over to Jamie and his friends, shouting, "You mother *fucker!*" so loud the whole bar turned around to look.

I threw the entire pitcher of beer in his face with one hand and slugged him in the jaw with the other. Sheer pandemonium broke out.

"Header! Header!" yelled Jamie in his French-Canadian accent. I kept on blasting him with every crazy piece of shit that came into my mind.

A very dramatic and satisfying end to the whole nasty saga, right? I could have just left it there, but I was an alcoholic, and my alcoholic brain demanded that I go way over the top.

Jamie tried to spit out his defense for ghosting me. *Keep going and order me a martini,* I demanded. Three martinis later, I started to play mind games. *How could I get him to REALLY pay for what he did to me, the hell he put me through?*

Ready? I made him take me to a club to dance and drink Cristal (hey, he owed me, right?), then I fell into bed with him. The next day, I kept him on the hook. We flew to the Bahamas and he bought me all sorts of expensive clothes. As I picked the shopping bag up off the counter, I had a real moment of clarity: *Heather, you are no better than a high-class hooker.*

I never saw Jamie again. If I did, I'd take the high road, say hello and move on. My behavior in that bar was a great example of how alcoholics think. Your thought process gets so distorted that you can come up with endless ways to make the most awful, pitiful, horrendous thing seem okay. That's how alcohol changes you: It takes you from being a good and decent person to one you don't even recognize.

· 5 0 ·

SAM, SAM, THE MARRIED MAN

Desperation was really setting in, and while I was falling off the cliff, I grabbed onto a branch: Sam, my married ex-lover. Brilliant idea, right?

I knew he was up in Maryland—not all that far—so I called him. He was happy to hear from me, and we made a plan to meet halfway at a hotel.

It was a just a couple hours' drive, not far but long enough to require some sustenance on the way. I had stashed some schnapps under the seat, drinking it all before I got to the hotel. Drinking, driving, drinking, driving. By the time I got to the hotel, I was fucking shitfaced! Sam didn't really understand why I was behaving so weirdly, but it didn't matter. We fell into bed, where I immediately started to throw up. Yep, not feeling very sexy at that moment. Ha!

After that night, I felt dirty about sleeping with Sam but still didn't have the sense to get out of it. It had been off and on (mostly off because of Jamie) for a year. Sam said he had to get back to Maryland, and I threw out the possibility of going with him. I had a friend there I could stay with.

"My wife is there, and it's a small town," said Sam. "Word gets around fast, and it might be a little hard."

"But you like it hard!" I said, and we both broke down laughing.

So I followed him back to Maryland, despite his little protest. Along the way, we stopped at an oyster bar and got a hotel room. The next day something changed.

"All right, here's the deal, Heather," he said in a real low voice. "You need to go back to Virginia Beach because I gotta get back to my life."

And I was like, "No, you don't. No, you don't." That sounded so needy, but I thought I could convince him not to break things off. *You know about the power of the pussy, right?*

(I can't believe I even said that, because it's so rude. My mother must be rolling in her grave, reading the words of her foul-mouthed daughter.)

He left. I followed him, but he didn't know I followed him. My daily routine became stalking him and watching where he went, even watching him meet his wife and kids. What the hell? It was like my conscience disappeared. *Why the fuck are you doing these crazy things, Heather?*

Because I wanted what I wanted, and I deserved to have a good life. I felt justified. I deserved it because my heart had been ripped out by Andy and Mark and Jamie and Sam, and I was just starting to *feel* again. Now I wanted what I wanted, and I realized that a married man was not going to fill the bill. I left Maryland and never saw Sam again.

· 51 ·

Same Shit, Different Day

After about 10 days, I knew I had to figure something out. I had to find a job, so I answered an ad in the paper for a job at a gourmet store. I knew the owner, and he was a bit of a hard-ass, but I had to do something. Dean was looking for a new catering director for his gourmet shop.

My interview was actually going to be with the chef, who told me during the first minute I was there that she was about ready to leave her position. She was asking me so many crazy questions and then she gave me a homework assignment: Put together a party menu that will blow her socks off. *Well, OK.* I silently wondered why she was so eager to leave her job.

All my stuff was still in storage, so I went to a bookstore and looked at a bunch of fancy cookbooks and all kinds of magazines to get ideas. Not that I had ever made any of those things, but I had to make an impressive showing or I was not going to get the job I so desperately needed.

Dean called me in for a second interview. He read over my résumé and told me I was the highest qualified person they had ever hired. The job would entail long days, which didn't matter because I didn't have a life. I was ready to work hard.

"I'm going to pay you the most I've ever paid anybody," said Dean. I was thinking that was pretty awesome. Back then, I was making like $65,000 a year, which was very good money. I didn't have anything to show for it because I had spent it all on partying. (At one point I flew a friend over to Spain, which is another crazy story with a lot of absinthe involved.)

So Dean was going to top that? Wow!

"We'll start you at $25,000 a year," he said, smiling. He thought he was really breaking the budget. I was thinking, *Fuck, how am I going to live on that?* I was used to spending like $500 dollars a weekend at the bars. Would that even pay for an apartment? Anyway, I jumped into it because $25k was better than $0k.

It didn't take me very long to start drinking at work—and hiding it, of course. Taking nips out of the cooking wine in the walk-in was my specialty. You know, I was pretty good at holding my liquor and my tolerance level had gotten way, way high. Not bragging, but I could drink a whole bottle of wine and be just fine.

Thankfully, I had a really good young crew (a lot younger than me) to work with, and they were just as fucking crazy as I was. We did these big events and would knock people out with our food. Everyone loved us. But it was getting harder and harder for me to keep up with my job because of my drinking.

On the home front, Amy and Bill were wanting their privacy back. Of course, you know, guests and fish start to smell after three days and I had been there way longer than that. I got cut a little slack because Amy was such a good friend.

Just at the right time, a friend of Amy's was going to be out of the country for a few months and needed a house sitter who could also look after her mother-in-law. The MIL lived in the guest house—by the pool. OK, so that would be easy. I'd have a car to drive and everything. My routine became: go to work, come home, drink. Lather, rinse, repeat.

Somewhere in there I started dating a guy from Suffolk named Philip, who I met at an outdoor festival in the next town over. We met in the beer line; how appropriate! Pretty soon I was doing the 45-minute drive back and forth to his place.

Philip was hot, like wrangler-cowboy hot, but he was as dumb as a box of rocks and arrogant as fuck. But he was a good lay... I mean really, really good. So my routine morphed into: go to work, go to Philip's, drink, have sex, and come home the next morning.

There was a reason he didn't come to "my" place, and that was because the owner said "absolutely no overnight guests, or parties, and #1 above all: don't drink the schnapps." Her precious schnapps was shipped to her from Ireland, and she kept it in the freezer. That was the last thing she said before she left: "Do not drink the schnapps!" Well, did you really think I was not going to start drinking the schnapps?

· 5 2 ·

THE SECOND DUI

One of those nights driving home from Philip's (drunk, of course) I decided it would be a good idea to have a nip for the road. The schnapps bottle fit nicely under the seat and was within easy reach.

Just as I was coming off the interstate exit ramp, this guy stopped in front of me and I rear-ended him. *Oh, God, no.*

He got out of his car, I got out of my car, and I was scoping his bumper for damage.

"Hey, look, there's no damage. We don't have to call the police or anything. We really don't," I said, with a lot of pleading in my voice. I could not get another DUI.

"Well, you scratched my bumper," he said. I went into desperation mode.

"Please DON'T call the police," I begged. "Please don't. Please don't, I'm begging you." As I was saying the last "please, don't," the guy called the police. He was such an asshole.

The patrol car pulled up not long after that, and it took about four seconds for the cop to say, "You've been drinking."

Like the smart ass I was, I said, "Ha! Not lately!" *Oh, Heather.*

He asked for my license and registration and then told me to move my car off the exit ramp, where he gave me a breathalyzer test.

That one was a .35, waaaay over the .08 limit.

And so I went to jail, which I don't remember. Somebody bailed me out, but I don't know who. The judge said I had to do AAC (Alcohol Awareness Classes). I hired the same lawyer who took care of my first DUI in 1985.

Because I blew such a high number, I had to do more classes the second time around. I shouldn't drink and drive; I knew that.

But at that point in my life, I was just drinking and drugging and it was just, you know, what's the big deal? After that little adventure, Philip and I broke up (not sorry, Phil).

· 5 3 ·

MOM

Every once in a blue moon I would have a clear thought and wonder why I was overdoing it with all these substances. Other people did it to numb some kind of emotional pain they had, but because I had convinced myself I was always the "happy girl," I was just denying my own pain. I finally figured out that I really started sliding downhill after my mom's death.

1991 was the year my mom passed away. My father had died from an alcoholic relapse nine years before that, when I was 21.

I'll never forget how I found out about my mom. My sister Elizabeth came knocking at my door in the middle of the night, crying and all red-faced. *What was wrong?* It had to be bad. I thought something awful had happened to Elizabeth, but I was about to find out that something awful had happened to somebody else.

"Mom's dead," she said through her sobbing. I think I asked her what happened without even knowing I asked her.

It turned out that Mom had a heart attack. She had bronchitis and went into a coughing fit, and that caused her to go into heart failure. Unfortunately for her, she was on the toilet—pants around her ankles—when it happened. *Oh, my God, what a way to go!!! Hello!*

I hated that for her. Her death devastated me. I loved my mom; she and I became great friends as adults. We used to drink together, go to dinner, just fun things like that. She was happy about all my travels and always liked to hear about my latest adventures. I brought Mark home for my cousin Carolyn's wedding, and Mom adored him from the start. She loved how happy I was with him. She died not long after that.

Elizabeth and I got on the first flight we could book to Virginia Beach. We went straight to my mom's house, only to find it all locked up, windows boarded up, deserted-looking. The last I remembered, my two older brothers were living there while Mom spent a lot of her time up in Tappahannock with her sister and brother-in-law.

My brothers had stayed there scot-free. I thought they should have helped Mom out by paying her some rent. We had a lot of disagreements over that, which didn't make for the most harmonious relationship between us. It didn't look like anyone was living there now, so there was no way to get in. I called my brother and he didn't want us going into the house. *What the hell? I'm going in the house!*

As devastated as I was with the loss of my mom, now I had to deal with this fucked up shit! I decided to call a locksmith. I told Elizabeth that we could just sweet-talk him and tell him we locked our keys inside. Well, he bought it, and we got in.

The little two-bedroom place was a total wreck. There were ashtrays with hundreds of cigarette butts in them. There was mold in the sink. It was completely disgusting. We just wanted to get out of there.

But I wanted something of Mom's to remember her by, so we held our noses and went on a search mission. I had given Mom a signed painting for her birthday (or was it Christmas?) and there were a couple of other things I found. We got out of there as soon as we could.

Somewhere along the line, my brothers found out that we got in and they were pissed. I didn't care.

Mom's funeral service was up in Tappahannock, Virginia. I decided to cook for the wake. It kept me busy and helped me cope. That was my outlet: cooking, cooking, cooking. I was just going to cook my head off.

After the service, we were all sitting around, drinking and eating, but mostly drinking—and nothing good happens when all of the siblings were drinking.

I must have said something outrageous to one of my brothers and he got really angry, and that launched into a full-scale fight. It was horrible. Then Buff and I got into it over who was going to be the executor of Mom's estate. She didn't appoint one, probably because she didn't really have much of anything and didn't think she needed one.

Buff stood up and announced he was going to drive to Virginia Beach, go to the bank, and make himself the executor of the will. Mom had always wanted me to have her engagement ring, but Buff disagreed, and there was another fight about that. It was just an ugly mess.

You know, you hear sometimes death either brings people together or separates them... the whole experience just devastated me and set me on a bad roll for a long time.

I would just drink, drink, drink, and the older I got, the more depressed I got about her death. Working got harder. Getting up got harder. Holidays got harder. Mother's Day would come and I couldn't handle it. Then it was Mother's Day, Christmas, Flag Day, any holiday. It would just completely sink me into "victim mode." *Why? Why me? Why did I have to lose my mom?*

And so I stayed in my shitty diaper, a warm and cozy place, for a very long time until I hit the rockiest rock-bottom ever.

PART IV

RESTAURANT CAREER

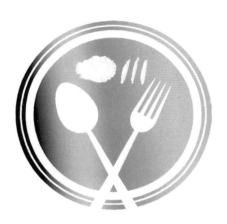

RAPE, RAPE, REHAB: RICH

Fast-forward to 1999. I was living in Virginia Beach again, rooming with a couple of black gay guys and four Great Danes. One of the guys was a waiter, and loved to dress in drag on his off-time. The other one worked for UPS. Then there was me, the crazy white girl in the middle.

That's when I started snorting meth—crystal meth—because one of the guys liked it, had it around, and knew where to get it. There was a dentist across the street from us who would exchange meth for "favors," and that got to be a thing.

Drag-Queen Waiter would say, "Come on, man (meaning me). Go over there and just slide him some sugar. We need some meth!" And I did it. That was crazy shit.

In the early spring of that year, I was walking on the beach and ran into an old high-school crush, Rich. Remember Rich, the rich kid? I never dated him, but I was always at his parties when his parents were out of town. I had to say, Rich was looking pretty good—and so was I, because I was tan from the Caribbean and thin from doing coke.

There was instant chemistry and all kinds of stuff was running through my head. *Oh, my God, you look so good, Rich! Did you know I was crushing on you in high school?*

"Hey Heather, you're looking good," he said. "We should go out sometime." I just melted. We made a date for that weekend. I was supposed to go to his house first for drinks.

It was spring, but it was early and still kind of snowy and icy. The roads weren't in great shape because Virginia doesn't get a lot of snow, so they don't prepare for it. Anyway, I drove to his house and we had drinks, as planned. He kept going to the bathroom, but I just wrote it off to the drinks. I should have guessed something was up.

We decided to go to a nice local restaurant, but I noticed he was really buzzed and probably shouldn't drive, so I did. He smoked pot all the way there. As soon as we got to the restaurant, I felt a shift in him. Rich was a former Marine, all hunky and hot. What I didn't know was that Rich was a *former* Marine because he had been discharged for psychological problems.

Dinner came and went, and then we had some more drinks. Rich suggested we go back to his house, but something told me I should just drop him off and go home.

"The roads are slick and I'm worried about you driving," he said. I assured him I'd be OK and not to worry. He insisted on me coming in, just to wait until it stopped snowing. So, OK, I did, still feeling like that was not the best idea.

Rich started pacing like a tiger. He made us some drinks, but even Heather, The Bottomless Liquor Pit was ready to call it and go home. By then it was coming up on one o'clock in the morning.

I don't know if Rich was doing pills or what, but he had gone to the bathroom (again) and came around the corner with his eyes looking really strange. I instinctively grabbed my keys and said it had been fun, but I had to go. I was getting nervous.

Halfway out the door, he reached around me and hooked me back into the house. He slammed the door, took my keys and threw them on the hallway table.

"Rich, dammit, give me my keys back. It's not funny," I said, trying to sound unscared.

"Try leaving and see what happens," he threatened. "The minute you get in the car, i'll call the cops and report you for DUI. You're not going anywhere."

Why the fuck would you do that? God, the messes I get myself into.

Then he started ordering me around, sounding like the Marine he used to be.

"Get in here. Now!" His tone had changed and he sounded downright angry. "Get over here. I mean it." *What the fuck?*

This guy was big. Much bigger than me, and really muscular. My stomach started knotting up. What else to do but have another drink?

"Get upstairs," he said, his voice lower than it was before. I refused and just kept eyeing the door.

"Get upstairs before I make you get upstairs, Heather." That was bad news. I turned away again and he grabbed my arm—hard—and literally started dragging me up the stairs, kicking and screaming. No one was gonna hear me because the house was set so far back from the street.

He dragged me into the bedroom and told me to get on the bed. I tried protesting, but nothing came out. He threw me on the bed and strapped one of my arms to the bedpost with his belt. *Was this really fucking happening?*

Then I saw that he had a knife, which he started twirling around and doing all kinds of crazy tricks with. Now I was really scared. The guy I was looking at wasn't Rich anymore. I didn't know who he was. *Was he having combat flashbacks, PTSD, what the hell?*

He started stripping, then he ripped my pants off and yanked my panties down.

"Now we're going to have some fun," he said. *He has a knife. I better just give in to this.*

That monster pulled me to the end of the bed, my arm stretched to the hilt. He kept playing with himself, trying to get it up, but he couldn't do it. He started rubbing against me to see if that would work. It was incredibly scary and horrible. *Horrible.*

No matter what he tried, he could not get hard, so he blamed it on me. "FUCK you!" He yelled, then he slapped me. I was afraid to blink. *How was I going to get out of this?*

Wait. He left my keys downstairs on the table.

He semi-passed out on the bed while I laid there, just frozen. Then I blacked out.

I woke up at five a.m. Rich was not there. Then I heard footpads coming up the stairs and I started shaking. *This is it,* I thought. *I'm done for.*

He opened the door and fell almost straight forward, onto the bed, and passed out. I still had my one arm buckled to the bedpost with his belt. *Fight or flight, Heather. Now or never.*

I listened for his breathing. "Rich?" The thought of him answering me was terrifying, but I had to make sure he was out, really *out.* I carefully, quietly undid the belt around my arm, so fucking quietly. My pants were at the end of the bed. *Forget the panties, just get the pants.*

I ran downstairs as fast as I could, snatched my keys off the table and heard a faint "Get back here" from the room at the top of the stairs. I ran like hell, literally jumped in my car and took off. I don't even remember where I went.

Maybe the worst thing of all is that *I never told anyone about that.* Not even my best friend Amy. I was so ashamed and so scared. I lived in fear of him finding me for a long, long time, but he got away with it.

Later, I'll explain how I came to terms with it. But until then, the shit didn't get much better. It got worse.

· 5 5 ·

Rape, Rape, Rehab: The Black Tornado Drain

Somehow, I was started working two jobs: one at UPS (gotten through my roommate) and another job at a cool restaurant down the block. I don't know how I did it. I'd have to be at UPS at four o'clock in the morning and work until nine. I'd start drinking before work—in the middle of the night, literally. It was only the good stuff: Grand Marnier. No drinking on the UPS job. Then I'd go to work at the restaurant and drink more, sneaking out to the bar around the corner and chugging drinks.

That period is a little hazy, but I do remember a couple of my friends from my yachting days (Gabby and Silja) were passing through Virginia Beach and wanted to visit. We met up at a restaurant around 11:30 a.m., and the first thing I did was order two Heinekens.

"It's so early, Heather, why are you drinking already?" Gabby asked, like these people didn't party all night when we were yachties. "Why not?" I snorted back. I think that alerted them that maybe I wasn't doing too well.

The next day they just did their own thing. I went and bought my usual medium-size bottle of Grand Marnier (the large bottle would kill someone) and polished it off before I went to work. I remember sitting on the edge of my bed, feeling very sad and gray, and thinking, *WHAT HAS MY LIFE BECOME?*

I was aware that I had become an alcoholic. I always said I would never be like my father. *And I was exactly like my father.* I had become a liar and a cheater and even a thief. Those are all things I never thought I would be, because I was brought up with values like honesty and trust.

Sitting on that bed, I had a huge vision of a big black tornado at the foot of it, pulling me down, spinning and pulling me down, trying to take me with it and sucking me down this nasty, dirty drain. I remember that like it was yesterday.

That was one of the many times I thought about suicide. *I can't do this! I don't know how to live anymore. I don't have a mom. I don't have a man.* I was the victim of everything; everything was always somebody else's fault. *Why don't I have this? Why don't I have that? Poor pitiful me.*

Instead of dealing with it, I would pour myself another drink and do some meth to wake myself up and make me feel "normal." When I went to work that night at the restaurant, I was full of alcohol and meth, feeling ten feet tall and bulletproof, as I am fond of saying.

My restaurant job was great because I could drink all day. The manager was a good friend, and so was the owner. Brett and Craig were very fair and very honest, good guys. They were just letting it slide, or so I thought.

One day in the middle of my shift, Brett walked over with this puppy-dog look on his face.

"Heather, you know I love you," he said. "But as much as it hurts me, I've got to let you go."

I couldn't believe it. He went on with his bad news.

"You're drinking at work, and I know you're sneaking drinks," he said. He could barely look at me. But instead of being mortified, like I should have been, I dove right into denial.

"No, I'm not. No, I'm not, Brett!" You know: *Deny, deny, deny to the end.*

Brett stood up and said, "We've watched you, Heather. The bartender has watched you sneak so many drinks. You need to pay for them."

I promised, swore up and down, that I wouldn't do it anymore, which was a complete 180 from "I didn't do it." I looked like a fool. Brett told me he couldn't keep me because I had become a liability. He apologized again and again, and suggested that I get some help. That was Brett.

I will tell you that I immediately went home, drank a whole bunch more Grand Marnier, and probably called the drug man. What I didn't tell you is that not long before I got fired, I was date-raped. Again.

A week or so earlier, an old friend-crush (Jake), had come into the restaurant. We started hanging out a little, then a little more and eventually it was like, "Let's go do some coke."

I just lived just across the street, so we went to my house and we started drinking... and drinking. Then this guy started turning on me, getting a little angry. We were in my bedroom and he got up and locked the door. It was Rich all over again.

I said, "Jake, I think it's time for you to leave." I was not going to put up with this again.

"Nope," was all he said. Jake was a lot bigger than me and he was starting to scare me.

After telling him a couple of times that I was tired and wanted to go to sleep, he started looking at me with this psycho leer.

"I'm not leaving," he said. "Not until I get what I want." And he raped me. Then he left. Just like that. The details don't matter; it was just as horrible as the first time. I was so ashamed of it that I didn't tell anybody for years. Both of those situations—Jake and Rich—created more victimhood for me. *Why did this happen to me? Why? Why?*

· 5 6 ·

RAPE, RAPE, REHAB: HEATHER, INTERRUPTED

It's funny, though, how the universe works. After trying to drink away the rapes and getting fired, my yachtie friends Gabby and Silja had apparently gotten in touch with Amy, my best friend, to express their concerns about me ordering double Heinekens before noon. Amy was already well aware of this and had been gradually pulling herself away from me. She had a little baby (who is my godson) and had better things to do than hang out with druggie-alcoholics. Many years later, she confessed that she couldn't stand to witness me slowly killing myself, so she pulled away.

Amy tried everything she could to stop me from drinking and acting like an idiot. I was 38 and acting like I was 15. But I was in the middle of this disease and felt like I didn't really have anything to live for. I was single, I wasn't hurting anybody else, so what was the big deal? I rationalized my drinking like that for a very, very long time. I didn't realize that other people were watching me go down that "black tornado drain."

One morning, the three of them showed up at my apartment: knock, knock, knock.

I opened the door and there they all were, just standing there looking at me. I was so tired, tired of my life. All I could say was "Hey, guys. Come on in." They filed in and sat down, like little kids in a fire-alarm drill.

"Heather, do you know why we're here?" Amy said. I was guessing they were going to take me out to lunch. Well, that was sure wrong. "We're here to do an intervention. You're drinking way too much and we're all worried about you."

After I picked my jaw up off the floor, I was surprised to hear myself say, "I know, I'm sick of it, too." They were expecting a fight from stubborn, headstrong Heather, but I didn't have any fight left.

They had already searched out a detox facility and they took me straight to it, that very minute. Those are some loving friends right there.

For 10 days, I had peace. For all of my drinking life, all I wanted to do was be at peace, and I had it at that detox place. I could sleep, I could relax. It was bliss.

In detox, they gave me Ativan so I could sleep, plus all the pizza I could eat. The irony of that was that eating pizza always made me feel fat, and I knew that if I ever felt fat, I was going to have to throw up. It was a bad cycle to be in.

(Wait: I forgot to mention another thing after my mom passed away—I became bulimic. For me that meant that every time shit hit the fan, I would throw up on purpose. I suffered from body dysmorphia, like a lot of people do. I'd look in the mirror and see nothing but fat, so I'd throw up to get those calories out of me. I was very surprised to learn in rehab that bulimia and alcoholism are very closely connected.)

On about the eighth day, I finally stopped shaking. My counselor recommended that I go to a 28-day rehab. There was no way I could afford that, but he said there was a state-funded facility in Portsmouth.

If you know Portsmouth, you know it's nice in spots, but the rehab place was in "the hood," the crappy section of town. I agreed to go anyway, and they gave me a list and told me to go home and pack a suitcase. I didn't know anything about rehab. I was thinking Betty Ford, tennis courts, swimming pools, people having fun not drinking. *Holy shit, was I wrong!!*

Of course, I ignored the list and packed like 15 pairs of shoes, all kinds of outfits, perfume, all the shit you're not supposed to bring to rehab.

Amy drove me there and dropped me off at Intake, right in the face of a very large lady. She opened my suitcase and started laughing. I didn't laugh back because I felt like shit, not having had a drink in 10 days. I was still pretty unstable and didn't really know who I was. I really didn't.

After she quit laughing, VLL (Very Large Lady) asked me what the hell was in my suitcase, referring to all of the clothes and little creature comforts.

"Well, I need outfit choices for when we go on our outings, and for all of the different activities," I explained.

She shook her head in some combination of amusement, disbelief, and disgust, and then proceeded to start taking my perfume, shoelaces, anything containing alcohol, and anything with a sharp edges out of the suitcase.

"Why are you taking my stuff?!" I yelled. She was so calm, like she had encountered this hysteria many times before. She pointed. "This has alcohol in it; that could be dangerous," she drawled. *Yada, yada, yada.* I just didn't care or have the energy to fight. I just went to my room, put away what was left and went to sleep.

The second day in rehab, they made us eat breakfast, lunch, and dinner. When you do drugs, you might eat something every other day, and when the shit wears off, you may go and get a taco or make some Top Ramen noodles or something. These people were making me stuff my face three times a day, and I was feeling fat, fat, fat. *Yeah, you know what, I can't do this anymore.*

All of the "inmates" had a monitor, someone who's assigned to keep an eye on you. On the third day, I got caught purposely throwing up all that food they were feeding me.

The monitor heard me in the hallway. "Are you sick? Why are you throwing up?" she asked. I told her all that food was making me fat, and when I felt fat, I threw up. *Oh, Lord, why would I say that? I busted myself.*

That bought me a trip to the counselor's office, where they asked me how long I had been bulimic, etc. etc. It came spilling out that it started after Mom died. I never felt worthwhile. I never felt pretty. I never felt good enough. I never felt like I fit in. I was constantly wearing a mask, a sad clown mask, which started when I moved from California to Virginia, 22 years ago.

I went on to explain that I figured if I could be really skinny, maybe I could get a boyfriend, and then maybe people would like me. Social approval, you know, that whole thing. In response, the counselor told me I was now going to be monitored 24/7, even when I went to the bathroom. No more throwing up. *Are you fucking kidding me? That's my go-to comfort thing. I'm battling addictions to cocaine, meth, and alcohol and you're going to take that away from me? Now shit is getting real.*

If you read that paragraph back, you will see how warped I really was during that time.

In spite of all these "deprivations," I have to say that as I went to those meetings and the group therapy sessions, things started to feel better. The rehab counselors helped me have closure with my mom's death.

I wrote a letter to her, telling her everything, telling her how much I loved her, and how sorry I was for the trouble I caused her. I had to read the letter out loud in group, and I was bawling my head off. It was very cathartic. I just cried, and cried, and cried myself out. I felt my mom there, and she understood, too. And then I burned up the letter. Then I forgave myself. I had it in my head that my mom left me because she didn't love me anymore. I finally understood that wasn't true. That little action "took."

The counselors also helped me deal with the rapes and got me to understand that I had nothing to be ashamed about. Those events were not my fault. The only thing I did wrong was to drink so much that I put myself in dangerous situations. But no one "deserves" to be raped, no matter how stupid their choices are.

That pain I had been carrying in my soul for so long created a very dark, open, gaping pit that I been filling with alcohol and drugs, trying to feel whole. After 10 days of detox and 28 days of rehab, I was feeling awesome.

On the day I was released, Elizabeth came to pick me up, and we went to a Ziggy Marley concert. Hysterical, right? I'm not supposed to be around pot or drugs or drinking. That stuff *never* happens at a Ziggy Marley concert, right? LOL.

· 5 7 ·

The Third DUI

After rehab, I wasn't quite sure what I was going to do, so I temporarily moved in with my sister. The counselors always said, "You need a way to plug in to recovery," to stay active in my own sobriety. They were always talking about doing things "one day at a time." Get a sponsor (which is like a sobriety mentor). Pray. By all means, go to the AA meetings.

Being all gung-ho to live this new sober life, I took their suggestions. I also knew a couple of guys I used to hang out with who were sober, so I thought, *Well, they're kind of cool, so maybe I can do this if I avoid bad influences.* I went to the meetings and hung out with sober people, but there was still something missing in me. I still had that empty, black hole. If you said something into it, all you would get was an endless echo, never an answer. Just a feeling of sadness, loneliness, and insecurity. I still didn't understand what that was.

But they said to just keep attending the meetings, and that will help you. I did go to the meetings and I kept coming home and still feeling lonely. I missed my best friend, alcohol. I didn't understand how people could live without it. I was sober and the drinking obsession had gone away some, but I wasn't happy. I missed my old fun self.

Anyway, the meetings did help me get to where I felt good enough to go back to work. Elizabeth worked at a restaurant down on the beach and helped me get a job there. I did my job, like any functioning alcoholic—we work 150 per cent to stomp down those demons inside.

· 5 8 ·

HOW TO BACKSLIDE IN 3 EASY STEPS

It was all looking good on the outside. After four months or so, I started building my relationships back. People were starting to trust me again, like my brother and sister-in-law. But the truth was that I was just kinda going through the motions. One day, as I was reading the AA Big Blue Book, I decided that it would be OK for me to have an O'Doul's, the non-alcoholic beer. It was hot outside and I really wanted a beer. *Yep, an O'Doul's will be all right.* So I went and got a six-pack, and in perfect alcoholic fashion, chugged like four in a row.

I kept thinking about the AA meetings, and how they helped, but they didn't help because I still felt like I didn't fit in. Maybe I wasn't participating enough in the meetings? Then I had a brilliant idea: What if I just did a shot of Rumple Minze (high-powered peppermint schnapps) before my meetings to loosen me up a little bit, and then I can really engage in the conversations, and absorb what I need to hear? Man, I was a champion rationalizer.

So I did shots-before-meetings for about a week. They probably all knew, but I told myself they didn't because it was peppermint, so people would just think I was chewing gum or something. Well, of course, anyone who's in AA can smell alcohol a mile away. I wasn't fooling anybody.

The next step in my rationalization was if people knew I was drinking, why hide it? I decided I was just going to drink. Yay, I'm going to have some fun again! I had a bottle of wine stashed away; I was going to go get myself some cocaine and do everything I haven't done in months. *You know, go hard or go home!*

I went out and went whole-hog, drinking shots and everything else all over town. Around two o'clock in the morning, I was still in party mode and made a call to a bartender who was a "friend with benefits." I hadn't done that in a long time. He had some drugs, so I drove (bad idea after having a DUI not even a year before) to meet up and hit the jackpot that night: booze, coke, and booty!

After partying myself out, it was time to get home. Instead of taking a cab, which

I should have, I was shitfaced, driving home, you know—one hand over one eye, one hand on the steering wheel. I think I heard somewhere that God looks after drunks and babies. Well, thank God for that. *Yeah, Jesus take the wheel!*

About 50 yards away from my driveway, I heard the siren and saw the lights in my rear-view. That yanked me out of my stupor in a hurry.

I'm being pulled over. Fuck, fuck, fuck, fuck. Crap, my house is right there. Do I run for it? Just jump out of the car, throw the keys on the ground, and run inside?

Somewhere in my blurry brain I reasoned that I might get shot at for doing that, so I stayed put. The officer came up to the car and asked for my license. Well, I didn't have a license because it was revoked for a year after my second DUI. I think the anniversary of that was the next day. That's how fate was rolling for me in 1999.

"OK, then I'll need to administer a breathalyzer," said the officer, who had a look on his face like *This is going to be such an easy bust.*

I blew well over .30 and couldn't pass the sobriety test. I couldn't walk two steps without falling off the line.

"That's it," said the officer. "Let's go." I pleaded with him to just let me put my car in the driveway and not leave it out on the street. He said that just in case I didn't get it, I was drunk and could not drive. My car was going to be towed.

"But I don't want my car to be towed," I said, unaware that I was not helping my case. "Can't you just put me in your car and take me home? How would that be?" I was pointing to my house to show him how close it was. I was bargaining, begging, pleading, just trying to get out of what I knew was going to be another huge mess of my own making.

"No," said the officer, slamming the door shut. "Your car would be towed anyway because I see you have a prior DUI." I tried again to get the cop to just let me go home.

"We're going to the jail," he said in a really stern way. O*K, so now I'm pretty much fucked. Another DUI, another night in jail.*

You'd think I would get it after three DUIs, but no. It set off a really bad drinking and drugging streak, one that should have killed me. After a few weeks of binging drugs and alcohol, it was time for my court appearance. It was not pretty. The judge looked at the papers, then looked at me, then at my lawyer.

"There is no lawyer on Earth who can get you out of this one," he said, glaring at me over his bifocals. "Your BAC (blood alcohol content) was over .30 and you've had another DUI within the last year. You were supposed to be staying sober. You need some jail time." My stomach started that familiar rolling feeling.

"What?!" I blurted out. "Wait! Can't I do community service?" You know, back to pleading and bargaining.

He wasn't having it. "No. You will do six weekends in jail. You will show up at the courthouse at seven o'clock each Saturday morning and you will be put in a holding cell until five o'clock that day. You will do that every Saturday and Sunday for six weeks."

And I was like, *Holy shit.*

Then on second thought, I was thinking, *How bad can that be?* I'll just bring a book. You know, bring some cards. Me, I was always thinking of a happy solution in a shitty situation; that's what I always do.

· 5 9 ·

JAIL TIME

So the day arrived... the day I started my jail journey.

I was a little hesitant because I wasn't quite sure what was going to happen: fear of the unknown, you know? I arrived at the jail like they told me. They cleared me through, checking me to make sure I didn't have any contraband on me. *If only!*

The guard walked me to my cell, where I came upon five very large gangsta-looking women. They looked like they could beat my ass to a pulp in one second flat. It was like walking into school and you're the only kid that doesn't have a "group." They were all checking me out like it was *Orange Is The New Black* or something.

There was also a scrawny little whacked-out thing who looked like she'd been on heroin for years. Just a little girl with stringy hair, sitting in the corner wearing a flannel shirt and jeans in the middle of August.

Because I'm the person who always tries to find that happy solution in a shitty situation, my mind leapt into action. *Holy crap, this could be my end. But wait: they're here. I'm here. What good is there in this bad situation? How am I going to get through this day and come out of it alive?* Hmmm, not much was coming to mind.

I quickly accepted the fact that I was the "new meat." I walked into the cell, all friendly, and said, "Hey, what's up?"

Dead silence. Blank stares. Just scowls all around, even the little strung-out white girl in the corner. She didn't even acknowledge me. She simply didn't give a shit.

Plan B was going to be necessary here. OK, let's bring fucking Crazy Heather out and see if that works. So I started talking like I was from the hood, like, *SUUUUUUUUUUP? Hey girl, how you doon?*

They all looked at me like, *Who the fuck is this little white-ass girl? She thinks she's all that.*

I just started spinning around in circles, as fast as I could, spinning and spinning, laughing at the top of my lungs. Just as that was getting their attention, I threw myself against the wall. *That'll get 'em*, I thought. *That'll make 'em think they do not want to fuck with this girl.*

I did a dead-stop and looked around, waiting for a reaction. The bunch of them just stared at me, wondering what I was going to do next.

"Y'all bring anything to drink in here? What's happening, girlfriends? How are we going to get some drinks in here? Let's get our drink on!!!" I was screaming through the bars.

"Bitch, we in jail." They just stood there. I knew we were in jail, *duh*.

"You been here before? Well, I ain't been here before," I said, going for the sympathy angle.

"Girl, just set down," said the biggest of the Big Girls.

"What do you DO in here? We can play cards, yeah? Don't they have board games?" The looks I got in response make me laugh now. They really did think I was nuts.

The second-biggest girl spoke. "Fuck you. There's no games in here. We just got to sit here on these floppy-ass mats."

That got me wondering about sleeping. Where were the beds? There were none, just those "floppy-ass mats." Somebody volunteered that you don't get the luxury of sleeping. It's a day-jail.

I started my crazy spinning thing again, laughing extra-loud, looking like the Tasmanian Devil, if you all remember that cartoon. By then, I was thinking that all of the Big Girls and Skinny Girl were right: I was fucking crazy. I threw myself against the wall and landed on a mat.

"My name's Heather," I said. They weren't sure what to do. And that was my first hour in jail.

For the rest of the day, we just all kind of kept to ourselves. At five o'clock, I was done. "See y'all tomorrow," I said as I waved goodbye, smiling at them. Thank God I had a bottle of vodka stashed under my car seat. (I was allowed to drive, but only to and from work, and to and from my jail weekends.)

That whole day did a number on me. I thought, *Shit, that was the longest day of my life. Maybe I'll take some Nyquil with me for tomorrow so I can sleep through the whole day. That's a good idea.*

Sunday morning, after the guard confiscated the Nyquil at check-in, I walked in to a little more receptive group. "Hey, man! What are we going to do today?"

"Damn, you're fucking crazy, girl," said the Biggest Girl. I started to spin around again, spin and spin until I got dizzy and threw myself against the wall.

"Goddamn! Why you in here?" she asked. "Judge wanted to teach me a lesson," I said. "I got a DUI and had another one too soon."

That must have struck a chord with them, and all my fellow homies started talking about why there were incarcerated. One girl was in for burglary; one in for beating the shit out of people and drug possession. The strung-out girl was like, "I don't know." She didn't speak much.

We got served some shitty breakfast, and then lunch, which was white bread and baloney. You know what they say about being in jail—"three hots and a cot"? Don't believe everything you hear.

While we were not best friends or anything, we started to chat a little, started to co-exist a little. I got through the first weekend, and I was stoked! *This wasn't so bad after all.*

Monday, it was back to my bartending job. That place was a breakfast restaurant that went into lunch, usually not a good money-maker, but it was good for me.

My specialty was frozen drinks, and we served a lot of them. One for the customer, one for me, maybe with a little shot of tequila on the side. *Who wouldn't love that job?*

The next weekend it was back to jail, do not pass go. I decided not to do the Crazy Heather thing this time around and they started accepting me a little more. Biggest Girl asked me what I did the past week. We were actually starting to become friends.

Being bored stiff is, well, boring. I wanted to see if we could get some playing cards. The other girls said it would never happen and they were laying bets on whether I could score some cards or not.

Because I was all "hood" by the second weekend, I was like, "Bitch, I'll get us some cards. Watch this."

About an hour went by and I knocked on the little plexiglass window for the trustee to come in.

"Hey, how you doing today?" I asked, in my nicest tone of voice. "You know, ma'am, we're here for eight hours, not doing anything. We've all become friends." (The girls are all smiling behind me. Funny as shit.) "Is it possible for you to maybe slide in a deck of cards? We'll be really quiet."

The trustee kind of looked at me, then at the girls behind me.

"Hold on a minute," she said. Talk about getting some respect from the girls!! The trustee came back in a couple of minutes and handed me a nice new deck of Hoyle playing cards. That was amazing. See, I made a shitty situation better. It's what I do!

After five weeks, those girls and I had become good friends. One more weekend, and I was done, so I told them where I worked and invited them to come on down and I'd buy them all a drink.

Damn, if not a week later, three of them rolled up to my bar. "Girl, you got some piña coladas for us?" *Oh, my God.* That was hysterical!!

· 60 ·

OLD HABITS DIE REALLY, REALLY HARD

That judge gave me jail time to rehabilitate me. Did that work? Ha! I got out and kept on drinking, and drinking even more. I ended up moving out of Elizabeth's place into a little one-bedroom. My life consisted of 1) work, 2) going to my favorite bar, The Tambo, to have a couple or five glasses of wine and hang with the owners, and 3) go home. (I was too broke to afford any coke then.)

One afternoon I went to an oyster roast with some friends, wearing a truly sexy shirt. It was a low-cut, short-sleeved, cropped thing with one button at my breast bone. Sexy, yeah. Put that with my cute low-rider jeans and I caught the eye of this guy.

"Well, that's the sexiest shirt I've ever seen," he said, not mincing one word. He had a super-buzz cut, almost shaved head. Glasses. Not real tall, maybe five-foot-nine. One of the funniest people I ever met. And he had the mandatory beautiful blue eyes, of course. Crystal blue eyes or hazel, those are my always my downfall. I just look at those eyes, and I see the twinkle and I think he loves me. *Deadly.*

"Well, thank you," I replied in a kind of teasy little way. You know, I always craved the attention of the opposite sex (because I never got it). I didn't think I was ever pretty enough, that I just blended in with the crowd, unnoticed. I was a great actress.

This guy and I were drinking beers with his friends, and he told me his name was Pete Farrigan. He asked me if I had ever worked at the Three Forks Diner, the place owned by my friends Brett and Craig—the place I got fired from.

I told him I had. "Gee, that's where I saw you. I was checking you out," he said, much to my pleasant surprise. "Want to go for a ride on my motorcycle someday?"

"Sure," I said. "Here's my number." *Hope springs eternal,* I thought.

After the oyster roast, I got a call from Pete, wanting to know if I'd like to ride down into the countryside past Virginia Beach. We could have some drinks, it'll be fun, he said. *Who am I to say no to drinks, ever?*

We went, and right in the middle of having a pretty good amount of fun, he told me he was married. FUCK. DAMMIT. I felt like I had come to a screeching halt at a big ol' STOP sign.

"Yeah, but we're really not together," he said. *Right.* I must be wearing a sign that says, *Hey, pick me because you're tired of your wife.* And you must have a tattoo on your forehead that says, *We really are together but I'm not going to tell you that because I want to get laid.*

It was too bad, because I liked him. He was funny as shit and very charismatic, not like anybody I had ever dated. So he dropped me off, all very innocent.

I saw him a couple more times after that (I know, I shouldn't have). He came over unexpectedly one night to find me drunk. So was he. And we hit the hay. *Oops!* There I go again, another married man. So pathetic.

It was kind of sad because I never looked at it like I was doing something bad. That's how sick and in a different reality I was then. I wasn't even thinking about his wife, or any of their wives or girlfriends. I was just getting what I wanted and I didn't have a conscience. I was just drinking and just doing whatever pleased me "because I deserved it." You would think that after what happened with Mark—all that cheating on me— that I would have gotten a clue. But nope, nope, nope.

I remember going to some big party at a famous local nightclub. Pete was there with his wife. One of the weirdest things is how I would run into these married guys out in public with their wives, but they never tried to bail. They'd even introduce me. Lucky I wasn't like Single White Fucking Psycho Female, trying to grab their husbands!

Pete knew I was moving into a second-floor place and offered to help. He had a friend (who owned a moving company) and they got all my stuff upstairs. Everything was in and the movers were gone, so there was nothing left to do but "christen" the new apartment. *Wink, wink!*

That little tête-à-tête did not last very long. The married thing just got to me. Maybe I was growing a conscience, after all.

Before we split, I asked Amy what she thought about Pete. She was like, yeah, he's really cute this, and really that, and everything else, but just FYI, he's married. Amy never judged me. She still doesn't. That's a good friend.

· 61 ·

FOR THE LOVE OF RUMPLE MINZE

Along with Tambo, I loved hanging out at the Pier 42 Grill. Great outdoor bar. I had crossed paths with a guy there several times in the afternoon and came to find out he owned the gift shop next door to the restaurant. My shot of choice at the time was Rumple Minze and it just so happened that this guy loved it, too. We got to know each other and started hanging out in the afternoons when business was slow.

His name was PJ Berglund. Huge, huge blue eyes, almost to the point of being kind of Gene-Wilder-like, but not quite.

One day he said, "Yeah, so I have four kids." I said I *didn't* have four kids, trying to be cute. He said he was divorced and that his ex lived in Maryland. *True? Not?* He told me was renting a room nearby, which I later found out was leased out by a friend of mine whose name was Cupcake. Yep, Cupcake. That was true, at least.

We started up a relationship, but I was very, very wary. I asked a couple of times if he was sure he wasn't married.

"I think I'd know," he laughed.

I explained that I had made that mistake before and didn't want to make it again. He repeated that he wasn't married.

"I'm not going to sleep with you because I don't know whether you're married or not. I'm not sure I believe you," I declared. "I'm trying to change my ways." He let it lie.

One night, late, we were sitting in his bedroom and he showed me what looked like a divorce decree (like I would know one if I saw one). That was good enough for me. We were having sex like rabbits and it was fun.

I remember walking down on the beach one night, full moon out. It was so romantic. I reminded myself that I was never telling anybody that I loved them ever again. PJ turned and gently grabbed me like he was going to kiss me, and you know what? He said, "I love you! I'm really in love with you!" My reflex reaction was to think, *Oh, that's nice.* Then I kept my promise to myself.

"You're not going to say it back?" asked PJ.

"This is so new... I don't know if I love you or not," I answered, seeing that left him kind of heartbroken. I had been burned so many times, I was just not going to jump in headfirst again. I was sticking to my guns.

PJ had joint custody, so his kids were around quite a bit. We got along great and I was a natural at taking care of them. One time they were at his place for the week and I asked them, "So let me ask you something Is it sad that your mom and dad aren't together?"

They looked at me with question marks on their faces and then they dropped a bomb, without even realizing it.

"Mommy and Daddy are together a lot. They sleep together when Daddy comes over," said the son, in the finest Kids-Say-The-Darnedest-Things style. I quickly put them to bed and found PJ downstairs.

It took about two seconds for me to confront him about my little chat with his kids. He denied it, swearing he wasn't sleeping with his ex.

I thought about what he said, then I thought about his kids. Sometimes, you know, I'd put the boy to bed and I'd go into his daughters' room and tuck her in, just dreaming about being a mom. I wanted it all: the husband, the kids, the home, the family. I always wanted that.

My brother and his wife had two kids who would just love it when "Aunt Poo" (that's what they called me) came to pick them up and take them on adventures. (I always aspired to be kind of like "Auntie Mame," if you remember that movie. You know, the cool, adventurous, awesome aunt who could teach kids all kinds of worldly things.)

We'd go down to the boardwalk, to the beach, to the State Park, and have so much fun. I love my niece and nephew so much.

One afternoon I brought them into Pier 42 one afternoon. I got a glass of wine and they ordered a Shirley Temple and a Roy Rogers.

"You guys can get anything on the menu you want," I said. "But don't get burgers and fries. Try something new." So of course, they wanted lobster. It made me happy that they took a chance and did something adventurous. It made me so prideful because I was a chef and wanted to open their horizons to awesome stuff.

Anyway, I was really into living the Mom life with PJ's kids. I would watch them when they were at his gift shop and take them on little adventures down on the boardwalk. Sometimes I'd ride with him up to Maryland when he dropped the kids off with their "real" mom. He'd leave me at a nearby Applebee's so it wouldn't be weird. I had no problem sitting in a bar by myself for an hour because I could always make a friend.

Thanksgiving came around, and we took the kids to Maryland. We had our own dinner and got to talking about Christmas plans. PJ had always managed (maybe he owned it, I was never sure) another gift shop up in Maryland during the holidays because it was such a busy time. He'd go up and work there a couple of days and come back and run the Virginia Beach store. That went on for all of December. He was really dedicated to his business and was trying to be a good dad to his kids. I couldn't fault him for that. And, you know, I thought, *Whoa, this guy's got a ritzy gift shop—maybe two—isn't he the shit?*

It was Christmas of 2000, and my whole life was PJ, wine, Rumple Minze, and work. It was fun and stable. He'd stay at my house sometimes, and it was really easy and really nice. Normal, you know. Not exactly the perfect family I was always wanting, but it was a pretty good substitute.

Then along came Dale.

· 62 ·

The Two Faces of PJ

One afternoon I was hanging out at Tambo, my nice dark, cool bar. Great atmosphere. It was all decorated for Christmas and it felt good to be there.

I always sat on "my" barstool—I must have worn a hole in it. I ordered a Rumple Minze shot, a glass of water, and a glass of wine. I looked over at the guy next to me, and he looked awfully familiar.

"Hi," I said. "You look familiar."

"My name is Dale," he replied, all nonchalant. Then it hit me, where I knew him from.

"Did you used to have the Blue Ray?" I asked. The Blue Ray was a local restaurant that was very popular in the '80s. Yep, it was him. He looked different; he had put on a little weight. Well, maybe a lot of weight. Then I remembered he had gone to jail for dealing cocaine.

He said, "Yeah. That was my restaurant." I complimented him on what a great place it was and tried to figure out how long it had been since I'd seen him.

"Let me buy you a drink," he offered. I always love to talk to old friends, find out what they've been up to. After we talked for about an hour, he said, "Hey, you want a bump?" He showed me his hand. I was like, "Absolutely!" *Why was it that people with coke always seemed to find me? Or did I find them?*

I went in the bathroom. I was greedy and did two big bumps, one right after the other, and came back out. Now we were *really* chatting. We sat there for a few more hours, but then it was time for me to finish my Rumple Minze and rollerblade on home. (Too many DUIs means you can't drive, so I learned to rollerblade.)

I kept running into Dale at different bars and we'd just hang out: good friends, good conversation, good times. He always had a lot of money and some cocaine in his pocket. I'm pretty sure he had a crush on me, but I wasn't interested. I had PJ, but I also liked having this new friend. FRIEND.

PJ informed me that he was going to be spending Christmas Day in Maryland with the kids and that Christmas Eve was reserved for me. I was so pumped! I went and got a Christmas tree and decorated my apartment up all nice. Each of the kids had a cool little present and PJ had a few things under the tree as well.

He left for Maryland two days before Christmas, saying he'd be home by two or three o'clock so we could spend Christmas Eve together. Then the deal was to go back to Maryland on Christmas Day and do that with his kids.

What nice plans we made! We were very much in love and had been seeing each other for almost a year. On the surface, everything was cool, but of course, there were some red flags. Didn't somebody say that when you look at someone through rose-colored glasses, all the red flags just look like flags?

I remember one day asking him, "Doesn't your ex-wife know we're dating?" He was like, "Yes, she knows."

So why couldn't I ever come to the house? I remember that time when the kids told me Mommy and Daddy slept together when PJ came to visit them. There were a lot of things I chose to ignore because I wanted what I wanted.

It was about 2:30 and he wasn't back yet, so I called the gift shop. PJ picked up.

"I can't talk now. I've got some work to do. I'll be home soon," he said, sounding pretty agitated.

Four o'clock rolled around. I called him again and had to leave a message. "There is a lot of traffic on the road and I don't know if you've gotten in an accident or not. Please call me," I said. Even to me, that was sounding kinda desperate.

Five o'clock. No PJ. I was getting worried and, of course, I was drinking a pretty hefty amount of wine as I was going down Worry Road. *Where the fuck was he?*

I called him again. It was about six o'clock. He picked up and sounded pissed off.

"Heather, I can't talk! I'm really busy!" Now he was downright angry. I kind of meekly asked him to call me back so I could at least know what was going on. Another hour went by. I called again. I never would have expected what happened next in a million years.

PJ answered the phone and didn't even give me a chance to speak.

"Heather! Goddammit, quit calling me! I'm not coming home. I'm not coming back there. I DON'T LOVE YOU, I NEVER LOVED YOU. And by the way, I'm NOT divorced!" Click!

That was Christmas Eve. Another man who had professed his love to me, then ripped my fucking heart out. It was like the movie *Groundhog Day*, only it wasn't one bit funny.

I wanted to know why, so I kept trying to call him back. He just turned his phone off. *What the hell just happened?*

The whole thing was just fucking devastating. I couldn't stop crying. I didn't know what to do. It was so fucking gut-wrenching. It was at that moment that the black tornado-drain started pulling at me. I just fucking snapped. I don't know if I lost contact with reality or what, but I didn't feel connected to anything anymore. Everything went dark and started boiling inside of me.

I picked my Christmas tree up, opened the door, and threw it down the stairs into the alley. Distraught, angry, so many thoughts and emotions were just flooding everywhere.

I promised those kids some toys, and now they're going to think I'm a liar. I can't believe he did this to me and to the kids. The kids loved me. I don't understand this. I hate him. I love him. I want to kill him. I hate my life.

· 63 ·

DALE

For the following 20 hours, I just sat there, staring at the wall. I didn't want to see anyone, talk to anyone, nothing. I just sat there. After a while I heard someone leave a message on my phone. It was Dale. I didn't want to talk to a soul.

He called again and I decided to pick up the phone. "Look, I can't talk," I said, trying to keep from crying. It didn't fool him because he said he was on his way over.

I barked at him. "Do not come over here. I mean it, Dale."

"But I have a Christmas present for you," he insisted. I told him I didn't want any fucking anything for Christmas. He completely ignored what I said and came over anyway, banging on the door.

This guy was like 6'4", you know, 300 pounds, a former football player. It was like the abominable snowman banging on a fucking matchstick building. My whole upstairs was shaking. The people downstairs were like, "What the fuck?" I yelled through the door for him to go away. He stood out there for a good half an hour, which he would never have done if he didn't think I was in a real bad place.

"Dale." I opened the door and said, "Go away." He pushed the door open and barged in.

He said, "I've got some beautiful presents for you." I repeated that I didn't want any fucking presents from him and told him to get the fuck out of my house. It felt like my skin was on fire, such a strange sensation.

He was like, "No, no, no. Here, do a bump, you'll be all right." I refused it. He kept insisting, in a sad pouty-lip kind of way. He would have done anything to be there with me at that moment, which left me feeling guilty and pissed off at the same time.

Finally I thought, *OK, I will do a bump and open the damn presents. Maybe then the fucker will leave and I'll feel better because I had some coke. Win-win.*

Out of the shiny boxes came two beautiful—and very expensive—dresses, and a pair of shoes that were amazing. Alligator heels. Very high-fashion.

"Come on, I'm taking you to a dinner party," he said. I told him I wasn't going anywhere. I had been crying for hours and looked like hell. I was in no mood to celebrate.

He just kept at it. "Come on, come on, Heather. Just have some drinks, some wine. Do the line, you'll be all right."

Because I always did what men wanted me to do, I put on one of the dresses, put on the shoes, and let him drag me to the party. All I remember is being fucking miserable while everybody else was having so much fun. There was drinking and caroling and holiday cheer all over the place, and I couldn't stand it.

Dale finally took me home and asked if I wanted him to stay over.

"Fuck no!" was my very rude response. No *goodwill toward men* for you, Dale.

After that night, I can honestly say that I just gave up on my life. Not thinking about suicide—but I was just spent. I was tired of never, never getting love and having my heart broken over and over again. I felt like there was nothing left of me and that I had nothing else to give. My emotions went numb and I fell into a bottomless depression, becoming a mechanical robot, and a broken one at that. I was in a very deep stage of *fuck everything and everyone.*

Dale kept calling and trying to get me to meet him here, meet him there. It looked like my life was going to be hanging around this guy who made me laugh, and that was going to be the extent of it. No love. So that's what I decided to do: Laugh, drink, drug, and have fun with Dale. That's it. As you might imagine, that was the start of another very unhealthy relationship.

I was still rollerblading to work and holding down my job at the restaurant. I'd meet Dale for happy hours, and we would just talk shit and have fun, all according to my plan. There was no attraction for me there. Dale was a friend and wanted to take care of me, which was fine, but there were not going to be any sexual favors. I was not going down that road again. I stuck to that, which was amazing.

Everybody always thought that Dale and I had a relationship because I became so co-dependent. I didn't see it at the time, but it was the definition of co-dependency. The more I hung out with Dale, the more I changed. It went by me because I was just paying my rent and drinking and drugging all the time, being that broken robot.

A year went by of me wearing fucking masks to fit into the various situations in my life. I would show up for holidays and dinner invitations with a bottle of wine in my backpack. I was never without wine or Rumple Minze. Some coke was in there most of the time, too.

The more of a habit that became, the more dependent I became on Dale. He knew he was holding the emotional cards, and if I wanted coke, it had to come from him (I didn't have the money), which meant I had to play nice all the time. Shame and guilt followed me around all the time, but I did what I had to do to keep that backpack well-stocked. Wherever I was, I'd take my backpack into the bathroom and chug my alcohol, do a bump.

I remember showing up at my brother Dink's place for a Christmas party once, and he had all his friends there. (Another situation where I didn't fit in, you know.) So I put my big bottle of wine in the fridge and drank more than anybody else, just so I could get some attention.

I feel bad now when I think about that because it was Dink's party, not a party for me. I think he was also pretty pissed off that I had a couple of my construction friends build a skateboard ramp for my nephew and drop it off in the front yard Christmas Eve. Did I ask Dink first? Hell, no. Heather did what Heather wanted to do so Heather could feel better. Me, me, me.

Proper people don't take their booze with them when they leave a party, as we all know. I guess I thought that excluded me because when it was time to leave, I grabbed my bottle out of the fridge. I could feel them all looking at me, thinking, *Who does that? Were you raised in a barn with a pack of wolves?* I knew how they felt and what they thought, but I just cared about my alcohol and people were starting to get tired of it.

My mother was probably turning in her grave, so embarrassed of the woman I had become. God bless her. She probably just shook her head at all the stuff I did. So sad.

Dink could clearly see that I had fallen off that wagon. He was so happy when I got sober that first time in 1999, because he was sober, too and he was doing well with his family and his kids. And that's one thing I always wanted, to have that good family dynamic, but at that time, I was only interested in what was in my backpack. That backpack was now my best friend.

· 64 ·

PEGASUS TAKES FLIGHT

One afternoon Dale and I were at an Outback restaurant (happy hour, of course).

Dale started reminiscing about his old restaurant days. He had always wanted to get back into the business.

"Why don't we open our own restaurant?" he said, and started doodling on a napkin.

"Cool," I said. "So how do two drug addicts and one massive alcoholic open a restaurant?" Then I realized he was serious.

I had no business opening a restaurant. My health was technically okay, but I didn't realize what I was starting to look like how I was acting. I wasn't getting invited to things anymore and couldn't understand why. I couldn't see that people thought it was weird that I was running to the bathroom every 10 minutes.

Of course, I was all in on opening a restaurant even though I knew virtually nothing about how to do it. Yet another bad choice. I left everything to Dale and just did what he told me.

In 2001, Dale bought an empty hair salon and along with me and some friends of his, turned it into a restaurant. We shopped all over at various warehouses, looking for stoves, fridges, and plumbing materials. It was only a 27-seat bistro, but you still had to do all of that.

The floor was just plain cement. Dale thought we should paint it glossy black. I suggested we square it off with tape, paint it black, and then paint a white checkerboard on top. We pulled up the tape and it looked amazing. *Oh my God! I accomplished that!* It was a small victory, but still something to feel good about.

We found some old church pews and covered them with fabric, a cool abstract pattern. There was an open kitchen that Dale was in charge of. I was "front of the house," and also the pastry chef, making all of the desserts. We had no dishwasher or freezer, just the basic Health Department requirements so we could be legit.

Our menu had veal, duck, lamb, and pasta on it. The restaurant became known for specializing in specializing. The nice, high-end clientele would come in and say, "I'm kind of on this diet, but like this sauce on the veal but I'd rather have shrimp."

So I would basically make a meal up at the table, then shout across the dining room, "Hey, Dale! Can you do a shrimp dish with the veal sauce, cut down on the butter and put some nice vegetables on the side?" I would put him on the spot so he couldn't refuse, so the answer was always, "Sure!" It really did make Pegasus a special place.

People also came for my chocolate pecan tart. I should have called it my "Paranoid Tart" because I was afraid of it; afraid it would make me fat. All you normal people, just enjoy.

CHOCOLATE PECAN TART

1 prepared 9" pastry crust
1 9" tart pan with removable bottom
8 oz. pecan halves
1 stick salted butter, cut into pieces
1/4 cup granulated sugar
1/4 cup brown sugar, packed
3 oz. GOOD bittersweet chocolate chips (60-70% cacao)
    or a good chocolate bar, broken into small pieces
4 large eggs
1/2 cup dark corn syrup
2 t. real vanilla extract
Pink Himalayan sea salt
Powdered sugar for a bit of a sprinkle
Fresh whipped cream

Preheat the oven to 375°.

Roll out the pastry, and using floured fingertips, put pastry in a tart pan and press into place. Use the rolling pin to trim the excess crust. Place crust in the freezer for 15 minutes, or until firm.

Prick the chilled crust and put the shiny side of a piece of foil down on the crust. Press into the edges. Fill the foil with dry beans and bake 15 minutes, or until it just starts to brown. Carefully lift the foil/beans out and bake for another 5 minutes more until the surface looks baked. Nobody likes a raw crust!

Cool the crust and set aside, but leave the oven on. Spread the pecan halves on a baking sheet. Cook for 8 minutes, regularly stirring, until they are aromatic.

In a large saucepan start to melt the butter over LOW heat, just to cover the bottom of the pan. Don't let the butter get brown. Add both sugars and keep stirring until butter dissolves. It should have a smooth consistency.

Add the chocolate and stir until it melts. Remove pan from heat and let the mixture cool to lukewarm.

Stir eggs into the lukewarm chocolate mixture one by one, followed by the corn syrup and vanilla.

Leave the tart on the baking sheet, and spread the toasted pecans evenly all over the shell, saving some for the topping. Pour the chocolate mixture over top and spread to the edges of the crust.

Bake for 25 minutes or until the filling is very slightly puffed in the middle and the pastry is browned at the edges. If the pastry seems to be turning too brown, cover the edges with foil. Set on a rack to cool.

Set the tart on a bowl so the outer ring falls off. You can either use a big spatula or two to lift the tart onto a serving plate, or just leave on pan and make do. Before serving I sprinkle the Himalayan sea salt on top just a little. The salt will bring out an amazing flavor. Sprinkle with the powdered sugar and serve with a dollop of whipped cream and toasted almonds, if you like.

<hr>

The restaurant, which shall be known as Pegasus, had a BYO liquor license. Customers brought their own wine, and the people who knew me brought two and gave me one for my "bathroom chugs." I finagled an arrangement with my drug dealer to be on a kind of delayed-payment plan, and he always got his money. People were enabling me all over the place.

The only thing I cared about was the next fix, the next thing. My soul was blank, full of nothing. People saw it in my eyes; the light was gone. That eerie, black tornado drain had sucked my soul out that Christmas Eve, and my only mission in life was to fill the hole with mind-numbing drugs and alcohol.

Anyway, word was getting around about Pegasus, and the food was amazing. We got written up by restaurant critics, and newspapers around the area were doing articles about us. We even got a nice blurb in a magazine. Tons of our friends came in to support us, and we took off. Yeah, I was a part-owner, but I didn't have a pot to piss in half the time and couldn't keep the electricity on.

· 65 ·

SWIRLING AROUND THE DRAIN

In 2001, I turned 40. My aunt and uncle threw a birthday bash for me, and my brother, niece and nephew came up to help me celebrate. I bought a really cool pink outfit for the occasion and felt like a million bucks. In my purse, I had lots of little miniature liquor bottles in case my aunt and uncle didn't have enough booze around.

I showed up on time—shitfaced—and stayed that way, all through dinner. I remember sitting at that big drop-leaf table and feeling like people were staring a hole through me, thinking, *She is so drunk and gross.* I was very thankful for the party, but I couldn't wait to leave and drink some more. Today, that memory makes me feel like an ungrateful bitch because my aunt and uncle aren't around anymore.

If you're reading this, *don't do that to the people who love you.*

I've come to terms with all this. As I'm talking about it right now and reliving it, I get an "ick" feeling because of who I was. I am not proud of that person. I had no dignity and no self-esteem, nothing. I was dead inside, just like a zombie.

My daily routine became awfully reliable. Most people have toast and coffee and orange juice, or a bagel, or cereal or something for breakfast. I had a half-bottle of wine. I didn't eat—can't be fat, you know.

I would go to work and wear the I'm-Just-Fine mask all through the dinner shift. *Welcome to Pegasus, we're so glad to have you. This fish entrée is the greatest. Yes, you're going to love the spicy remoulade.* The energy it took to do that was enormous. I was just a fucking mess, like a melted candy bar in the hot sun.

Every afternoon, I'd go buy four-packs of miniature Rumple Minze. By the time I left the liquor store parking lot, two of those would be chugged down by yours truly. Then back to work for the dinner shift.

"Right, Alice?" That's what one of my customers started calling me, like from *The Honeymooners.* He'd say, "Hey, Alice. You're going to the moon, you're coming down from the moon. Alice, come down!" He knew I was always high on something.

I drank all day and all night. I drank to the point where I had such a high tolerance for drugs and alcohol that I could be completely wasted and still function. I was out of control, but I could control it, if that makes sense. At two in the morning, the TV would still be on and I would be together enough to make sure I left a little coke and a little wine for the morning. If I didn't have it, I'd go into a full-blown panic, and who wants to start their day like that?

Dale and I were just bs-ing and he threw out this idea of going to a college football game at his alma mater (he used to be a defensive lineman). We could shut the restaurant for a couple of days and get out of town, take a break. He even had a friend we could stay with. I was thinking that was an awesome idea. I was a little bit worried about the idea of a trip with Dale because every once in a while, he would try and make a move on me. I would be like, *What are you doing? You're just my friend. You're my restaurant partner. Knock it off.* And then he would behave.

It had been a while, and I was excited to go somewhere new. Dale had a Jeep Cherokee that we stocked up with bags of coke and magnums of wine. We were loaded for bear!

I remember stopping at some rest area along the highway. Neither one of us saw the state troopers, who were right in front of me as I got out of the car and a couple of bottles of wine fell onto the pavement. (Luckily, they didn't break. That would have been the worst.)

Dale was yelling, "Mother fucker! Heather, get out and use the bathroom already. Jesus Christ!" I was a handful. I was just that girl!

We got to Dale's friend's house and went to the game. Everybody started leaving in the last quarter, but as true fans, we stayed—and our team won it in the last 10 seconds! The stadium, all the people... what an amazing experience, one of the best of my life!

Afterward, we went to some bars and cruised around town for a while. The next day I knew I was going to need some coke, and this was in the days before debit cards. I couldn't have a credit card because nobody would give me one, so I always had to write a check. There I was, writing checks I knew wouldn't clear because there was no money in the account. But I wanted a gram of coke, so I wrote a check to "Cash" for $50. More and more, I was turning into a liar, a thief, and a cheat. I was sneaking around, stealing Dale's coke because he would never remember what he did with it. Now I was writing bad checks.

On our way back, we came through some little town in Virginia late at night. Neither one of us could stay awake and we were all out of drugs, so we stopped at a gas station to sleep. *Ugh.* I remember feeling so dirty and gross and all I wanted was a Diet Coke.

So it was back to work for Dale and Heather. On the outside, the restaurant was all good. On Heather's inside, it was getting harder and harder to function. It wasn't like I didn't try to fix it. I went to detox to dry out and sleep for a couple of days. I got out and went back a couple of days later. Between 1999 and 2001, I was in detox five times, but it just wouldn't "take."

Maybe I was really insane; maybe a psych center was the answer. I thought I needed to do that because I didn't know how to live life anymore. After checking myself in and thinking this was going to be the big answer to all of my problems, they only kept me there for one day.

"You know, you're an alcoholic," said the doctor. "But you're not crazy. You just need to go to AA." *Yeah, that's not going to happen. AA didn't work for me before, ain't gonna work for me now.*

I used to have a journal (I still have it today). When I read it, it breaks my heart because of all of the sad thoughts I had when I was in that self-destructive shithole. I really didn't know how to get out. It was like looking up at the sky and being underwater in a pool. I could see the sun shining down through the water, but I couldn't reach it.

All I needed to do was just push off the bottom and break through the surface, but I just couldn't do it. I was drowning in my own self.

· 66 ·

The Rat Hotel

The restaurant was still going strong, but I came to find out that Dale's house was being foreclosed on because the restaurant profits were going up his nose and he wasn't paying his bills. I was so out of it by 2003 that I couldn't even get mad at him. He was drugging so much that he didn't care either.

I think he wanted to move in with me, but I was really sick of my old upstairs apartment and didn't want us living there. It had gotten so messed up because I was a drug addict and an alcoholic and cared way more about getting high than cleaning. I skipped out on my last month's rent and Dale and I moved into a rat-infested hotel downtown. *What a great idea!* My life was officially in the shitter now.

All my stuff had nowhere to go when I moved into the hotel, so I had to put it in storage. (No biggie that I didn't have the money to pay for that.) All of my pictures from when I was a little kid, trophies—all those things that mean nothing to anyone else, all the mementos that you treasure—got boxed up and put in a storage unit. There were pictures of my mom, things of hers and my dad's from my childhood, so many little things. The rest of my stuff—dresses, shoes, clothes—was in garbage bags at the hotel. I figured as long as I tried to look good, maybe people wouldn't see how fucked up I was.

Nostalgia would tug at me sometimes, and I'd want to go to the storage unit and "visit" my old stuff. It made me sad, thinking about the good old days, because I was *living* then. I wasn't living now; I was only existing and trying to put a shiny-happy face on it. I was like the Emmett Kelly clown, but I wanted to turn that frown upside down—I just couldn't. It was so hard.

The storage-unit manager called me after a few months and told me I had to come down there and pay for the unit rental or they were going to auction off all of my stuff. I got there five minutes too late. All of my belongings had been thrown in the dumpster because the auctioneer said they weren't even worth selling.

"Which dumpster? Which dumpster?" I was frantic, asking the manager where they had thrown my stuff. It was all I had left of my mom and dad. It was like my parents were being killed right in front of me.

"The garbage truck just left," he said. I was so fucking angry and so fucking sad. Heather gets screwed again. Me, the victim. It was never my fault. It was Dale's fault. It was the manager's fault. It was the garbageman's fault.

Dale would get the brunt of it, with me yelling at him that he had made me lose all my shit about every 10 minutes. He would just say, "Here, go buy some coke." He'd whip out some money and I'd call the drug guy. That was my solution for all problems.

I should mention that in the middle of the rat-hotel adventure I was taking care of Dale's parents, who lived right down the street from the hotel. Dale had gone to Key West to help some good friends of ours, JJ and Carrie, move there.

Carrie and I were great friends. I used to go over to her house and we'd watch *Absolutely Fabulous* (the British TV show featuring the alcoholic friends Edina and Patsy). We'd do our drugs, drink our wine, watch those shows and laugh our ass off, just like Edina and Patsy.

I remember being over there late one winter night, kind of icy/snowy. Carrie and I were walking outside and the next thing you know, we both hit a patch of ice. We slid down their stairs, off the deck, and into a ditch. The guys, who were watching football, heard a scream and came running out. We were laying on top of each other laughing our fucking asses off. The guys thought we were crying from being hurt. We didn't care because we were so stoned.

Dale closed the restaurant for a few days to help JJ and Carrie move to Key West, and he put me in charge of looking after his parents. That was good because I got a little break both from the restaurant and from Dale. I would go over to his folks' house at night so his dad wouldn't have to stay up with his mom. Staying up all night was not a problem for me!

Dale's mom was really sick, pretty much bedridden. I'd change her bed, clean her up, and we'd talk and talk. His dad was getting old and he was not in the best of health, either. It was easy, though, just as long as I had my wine and my drugs. (By then, it was all maintenance. Those things didn't even get me high anymore because I had developed such a tolerance to them.) I'd go over there and sleep on the floor. When I woke up at seven o'clock, I'd drink the wine and do the coke I'd left by my sleeping bag, then get up and take care of Dale's mom.

Dale returned from the Keys after a few days and reopened the restaurant. After roughly three years into it, I remember standing in the main dining area after closing one night thinking, *Where's my family? Where are my friends? Wait, I don't have any family or friends. What is wrong with this picture?* And then I realized that everybody had pulled away from me. The only people in my life were Dale and my drug dealer. Maybe Dale's parents. But they were just faces to me, like not even real people.

Not even Amy, my best friend, was a "real person" to me anymore. She still lived with her husband Bill in Virginia Beach, but she had pulled away from me, too.

She and Bill had gotten a hot tub, and she kept talking about this accessory she wanted for it. I thought I would get it for her for Christmas. I went over to her house, unannounced, and found her and her sister in the hot tub out back.

"Hey, how you doing?" I said. They basically just ignored me. Like a look of disgust or something. I remember trying to start a conversation, asking Amy what was up, what was she doing for the holidays. Nothing.

"OK, well, here it is," I said, and dropped the present on the patio. "Thanks. Merry Christmas. Goodbye." And I left.

*Whyweretheybeingsomeantome?*Thatwasthewayifeltabouteverything,likeavictim. Ithinkaboutthatshitthatidid.Man,howcouldijustshowupatpeople'shousesandknock onthedoor,like,*Hey, what's up? Just came to visit. Drop everything and pay attention to me.* I didn't realize that people were seeing what was happening to me, but I was not. I just thought if anybody was getting hurt, it was me. I still loved everybody, but everybody was not loving me. My life was really out of control. My coke habit was costing me about $300 a day, so I was constantly borrowing money for this problem, borrowing money to cover that debt, whatever. To pay someone, I borrowed something. It was robbing Peter to pay Paul. The bottom was coming, I could feel it.

· 67 ·

THE WHEELS START COMING OFF

In 2004, Dale was turning the big 5-0. Many of the restaurant patrons—people and investors who supported us (and partied with us) along the way—wanted to throw him a big surprise party. People came from his college; his dad came; we put photos from his old football days up on a big screen. It was really nice, but I was only half-there. Thinking back, I was never happy where I was. I could never live in the present moment and enjoy it. Always on the outside looking in.

Somehow, I finally came up with enough money to get out of the rat-hotel and find my own place. Got a cute little two-bedroom a block and a half from the beach! The best part: only $300 a month and five minutes' walk to work. (Still no driver's license.)

At the new place, I had a really nice neighbor, Nick. He had a beautiful two-story house that I would take care of whenever he would go away. My downstairs neighbor liked to play backgammon and do coke, so I became the friendliest neighbor ever!

Nick didn't do drugs, and he for sure didn't know that I was doing a lot more cocaine at my friendly backgammon games with the other neighbor. We started a little flingy fun thing, more like friends with benefits. I didn't realize that he actually had a girlfriend, who I met later on down the road. Again, all the good ones are taken—but even the good ones seem to be looking for something on the side. I've never understood that.

This new location gave me a little sense of calm. Nick and I would drink, lay in bed, watch TV. It was as close to normal as I could imagine. It wasn't *really* a good life, though; I was just trying to pretend that it was. The foundation was cracking, and other people were starting to see it. This girl I knew would say to me, "Heather, why don't you just leave the restaurant business? You're not happy. You're sad all the time." And, you know what? I was that girl. It was getting harder and harder to cover up my sadness.

In spite of all that, Pegasus had developed a really good clientele, not just because of the food, but also because of the Dale and Heather Show. We were funny as shit, really witty banter. The customers loved the good time we gave them every night. Yeah, well, that witty banter became vicious sarcasm, and it turned ugly.

About four years into the restaurant business, I remember having an argument with Dale over wine and drugs, or whatever. Pegasus had closed for the night, and it was just the two of us standing outside the front door, well after one a.m.

"Don't come back tomorrow, Heather," he said. For some reason, this wasn't a shock to me.

I was like, "No, I'm not leaving you to run this place alone. Give me my wine."

"Get out of here, Heather," he snapped. "You're becoming a pain and you're obnoxious." I thought maybe I had better leave because you never want to piss off a big, huge, Greek man. Not ever.

But I wanted my wine, so I put up a fight, like a stupid ass. I remember trying to push past Dale and open the door with him pushing back on me.

"Let me get the fuck in this restaurant; you give me what I want! I want my wine!" I mean, I was just crazy. He literally picked my ass up and threw me into the alley. I landed on my shoulder. *Oh, mother fuck, that hurt.*

"You'll never fuckin' see me again. Nobody puts their goddamn hands on me," I yelled. I got up, stalked away, and went home, crying and holding my shoulder all the way. *This is fucked up. I can't do this anymore. I am never going back there again.*

In the light of the next day, I had a clear thought: *You know what? I have to find something else to do.* I saw an ad for a design school. I wanted to be a designer. So I called to ask about the school and talked to a very nice man. The thought of going away to school in Maryland was appealing... but in reality, just another escape. *When would I ever learn?*

I actually thought very seriously about design school because at that point in my life, I had *nothing*. I just wanted to bail on it all. I was getting so paranoid living by myself, always thinking there was somebody in my house, or a man in the bushes. After doing way too much cocaine, I would think somebody was trying to break in and kill me. I lived in fear of just about everything.

In the end, I had to abandon the idea of design school because the money wasn't there. My landlord and I got to talking about changing careers, and he mentioned that bed-and-breakfast owners were always looking for people with good restaurant experience. Why not? I answered a newspaper ad for a place in Norfolk, about 30 minutes north of Virginia Beach.

· 68 ·

PART-TIME JOBS, FULL-TIME ADDICT

The B&B was a big old antique house. I walked into the foyer and spotted some port in a beautiful decanter with four little glasses on a tray. *Fancy... even if I think port is gross!*

The owner, Wayne, came in and introduced himself. Very polite and all. He wanted somebody to come in and make breakfast for the overnight guests each morning. It should have been a very easy job for me. Wayne and I hit it off and he hired me right there in his fancy parlor room.

That was a relief because now I had a solid excuse to give to Dale, who was sending employees over to my house, begging me to come back to the restaurant. I told them I wasn't coming back, that I had to separate myself from Dale and that restaurant or I was either gonna kill him or myself. I was serious about that. I couldn't fucking deal with it anymore.

They would lay a huge guilt trip on me. "Well, Heather, there's people that won't come in unless you're there," they would say. Because I am a lifelong people-pleaser, that got to me.

I said, "Well, you guys figure out who's not coming in, and if it's so and so, then I will come in. I will play nice, serve them dinner, and I will leave. And I will knock out the terms of that with Dale and then I will go home because I have got to get another job."

There was a little bit of enlightenment right there in my brain: *You have got to get out of this fucking dysfunctional cycle, Heather.*

I continued going up to Norfolk for Wayne's training sessions. He showed me what I was supposed to do, how the kitchen was organized, all that stuff. I remember him and I sitting in the kitchen one night after I'd been there a couple of weeks.

He said, "We got to go to Costco and get some stuff. We can eat a bunch of samples for free, then we'll come back and have a couple beers." That sounded like a plan. Then Dale called and asked me if I could pick up some of this special olive oil for him while I was Norfolk. Hey, I had a drug dealer in Norfolk, so I could knock out three birds with one stone.

Wayne asked what I needed to pick up. "Olive oil," I said, adding that "I might get a little 'whatever' while I'm there, too." That could have gotten me fired, but it didn't.

"Oh, my God," said Wayne. "Can you get me some?"

Fuck me. Now I'm working for somebody ELSE who likes to do cocaine! There is no escape!

Wayne seemed to be more stable than most, but people who do coke usually have some kind of fucked-up shit about them. I think he was gay but didn't want to come of the closet.

I remember he kissed me one night, but it wasn't like a real kiss. I was showering in his apartment and we got all lathered up and I was like, all right, time to get lucky. The next thing you know, he just got out of the shower. *What the fuck?* This guy was giving me so many different signals. Maybe he was trying not to be gay; I don't know. It was just par for the course in my love life.

Every day, I'd go back and forth from Virginia Beach to Norfolk, borrowing Dale's car and driving on a suspended license. I liked my new job and I wasn't doing drugs all day. I had a purpose, and it was making me feel better. But the minute I was done with work, you know, it was *game on.*

After about a month in, Wayne said, "Why don't we go down to the beach and party?" He had started flirting with me a little, but then he would pull back. It was weird, but I said OK. We got some drugs, went down to Virginia Beach, and got completely wasted, though we still had enough sense to know we couldn't drive back to Norfolk that night, so we just stayed at my house.

He said, "Well, we've got guests at the inn, so we're going to have to get up early and get back there in time for breakfast service. Set the alarm clock." I did, but set it for PM instead of AM.

We both woke up at 8:30. He was fucking pissed! We hauled ass back to the inn to find that the guests were in the kitchen, making their own breakfast. Wayne lied.

"My sincere apologies, folks. We were in Virginia Beach and the car broke down. I couldn't get it fixed in time to make it back for breakfast. I'm terribly sorry." He was a pretty easy liar.

Then privately, he blamed it all on me. *But hey, Bud, you were just as drunk and stoned as I was.*

So there I was in another crazy work environment and another crazy relationship with another crazy cokehead.

To complicate matters, I started working at Pegasus again—just a few hours a week. People kept asking where I was and why I wasn't there. I guess I felt obligated to be there. Got to please the people.

I remember on one of my Pegasus shifts that I'd run out of cocaine. I was waiting on tables in a full restaurant and suddenly the whole place started to spin. I couldn't breathe. *Fuck, I think I'm having a heart attack.* Everyone saw me gasping for air. Two nurses who were at the bar rushed over to take my pulse. My heart rate was insane.

One nurse yelled, "Give me a paper bag, give me a paper bag!" Somebody found one and they told me to breathe into it, like you see on TV. Well, it worked. I was breathing again.

"Don't worry," said the younger nurse. "We don't need to call an ambulance. She's just having a panic attack." I had never had a panic attack. Never. That was one of the lightning-bolt moments when I realized that I couldn't live without drugs and alcohol.

Drugs, alcohol, sleep, drugs, alcohol, sleep. A good day would be when I would meet a guy at a bar and then invite him to come to the restaurant. Dale would always cock-block me and make the guy feel so fucking bad that he would leave. Dale was like, "If I can't have you, nobody can." I was in a sexless marriage with a restaurant. It was nuts. Between Dale and Wayne and Nick, my life was full of crazy.

Dale was getting fatter and fatter and unhealthier every day. Finally, he had one of those surgeries where they do something to your stomach and he lost like 150 pounds. His whole demeanor changed, and that was a welcome thing.

He wanted to go to the beach in Florida because he wasn't embarrassed of his body anymore. So we drove to Palm Beach, got some cocktails, and sat on the beach. It was awesome. Dale had hit his goal, was eating much healthier, and wasn't drinking as much. There was that brief period where things were kind of normal-feeling again. But like I said, it was very, very brief.

I remember the bright times, when I had to get flowers to take to the bed and breakfast. People in my area had beautiful, beautiful gardens. Everything was overflowing with beauty. I felt like a little girl in the country.

I'd take a basket and go around the neighborhood very early in the morning, cutting fresh flowers. Then I'd bring them up to Norfolk and put them in the vases on the tables. That was one of the things that made me feel really good. It didn't even occur to me that I was stealing those flowers from people who had worked hard to grow them.

One day Carrie (my AbFab friend) called me from Key West. "Why don't you come down here for a couple of days?" she said. I took her up on it and flew in, all fucked up, to Key West. I loved it. There was a ridiculous amount of drinking going on down there, and people were so nice. I stayed for a couple of days and had to pull myself away. I thought, *Oh my God! This is paradise. This is the most amazing place ever.*

Then it was back to reality, back to the restaurant, back to the B&B, back to existing. Something had to change.

· 69 ·

LAST DAYS

If you've gotten a sense that my life was spiraling down... down... down, then I have done a good job in telling my story. The crazy addictive lifestyle I was living was taking me to some pretty scary head spaces.

Instead of going back to Virginia Beach after work one night, I decided to go into Norfolk and get some drugs instead. I wound up meeting somebody other than my regular dealer and was directed to go to a skanky place that was not in one of the nicer areas of town. But I trusted them because my guy knew them. I rolled up to the house, and they were actually pretty nice and invited me in. A lot of other people were hanging around; some snorting lines, some smoking crack.

I started doing some lines, watching how shitfaced everyone was, passing around joints, liquor, whatever. Some people were shooting up. I didn't think anything of it. I was just a skinny-ass white girl in a crazy-ass situation, and I thought it was perfectly normal for me to be there.

After alternating lines of coke with smoking some crack, I lost track of the time. Maybe a whole day went by, I'm not sure. I woke up and there were people strung out everywhere. It was like a scene out of a junkie movie. Some people were crashed; some people had been up all night drugging and they were all bug-eyed. *Fuck, is this really my life? I could have been killed.* That last couple years of my fucked-up existence, I put myself in some pretty crappy predicaments. I thought I was indestructible. I really didn't care. I really didn't. I was losing weight, obviously a sign of bad health, but I thought I looked good. Nice and thin, you know.

I grabbed my coke, grabbed somebody else's, got a cab, and went home to a bunch of angry phone messages from Wayne, wondering where the fuck I was. Luckily, I didn't have to work that day, so I just crashed on the couch and ignored him.

Not that I didn't know it was coming, but Pegasus finally closed in 2005. I think we sold it for five dollars... maybe it's a taco place now, who knows. Up until then, I was in there maybe once a week, trying to schedule whatever hours I had so I wouldn't be around Dale.

He had become so controlling over me, and I allowed it because I had given up on myself. He was the puppeteer and I was the puppet. I was now taking care of his parents at night, even when he was in town, sleeping on the floor, drinking my wine the minute I got up, and going back home to my shitty-ass apartment.

One of the last times I worked at Pegasus, Dale came in unexpectedly. He walked in the back door and came right up in my face.

"Heather, my dad's missing a lot of money," he said. *OK, so why are you telling me this?* I asked him what he meant.

Dale said, "He hid a lot of money in his garbage disposal and now it's gone." It was pretty clear that he was accusing me of taking it, which really pissed me off. I stomped out of the restaurant and went over to his parents' house. His dad was sitting in the kitchen.

He said, "Heather, where's the money?" I was dumbfounded. "What money are you talking about?"

He said, "I'm missing six thousand dollars."

I was like, "Well, I don't have it. Look at me, do I look like I have six grand laying around?"

He asked again. "What did you do with the money?"

I said, "I didn't take your money. Give me a polygraph test. I don't know where the money went, but I think your brother took it." *Who hides money in a garbage disposal anyway?*

After that, I didn't take care of Dale's parents anymore because his dad didn't trust me. That really hurt my feelings because I had given a lot to those people, taking care of them because nobody else would. Dale's brother would pop in from time to time, but he never said much because he didn't like me. Maybe he thought I had him pegged.

Dale and his brother had a really crazy relationship. Dale did something very nice for his brother that a lot of people didn't know about, and it pretty much saved his brother's life. But we'll leave it at that, because that's not my story to tell. His brother has to live with that, and with stealing his dad's money.

Dale's father has since passed away, and so has his mom. I wasn't allowed to go to the funerals because they all thought I stole that money. I don't know if they ever found it.

I kept telling them to give me a polygraph test, but they never took me up on it. Well, I guess it's easier to blame me than to find out the truth.

Dale talked a lot about moving to Key West, an idea I liked because he would be out of my hair and I could just work for somebody else. He eventually made the move, which was good in some ways, but it pulled up my only anchor. As messed-up as it was, he was still my only anchor.

That started me drinking more than ever because Dale wasn't there to "check me." I constantly had liquor in my backpack, bottles full. I was rollerblading all over town with full bottles of liquor on my back. It was amazing that I never got hit by a car.

Eventually I was nicknamed Roller Girl because I'd always go rolling into my favorite drinking hangouts, Tambo and Pier 42. I'd hook up with different people just to fill that empty space in my soul. But every "morning after," I would find that empty space still there. I wondered why everybody always had so much more than I did, and how did those people get so lucky? It wasn't fair that I didn't have parents or love or clothes or a house. All I had was sad.

Meanwhile, my brothers Chris and Buff were living together a few blocks from me. We had a bit of a strained relationship. I was in my own hell, and they were evidently in theirs. They liked to smoke a lot of pot and even deal a little.

My brother had a couple of daughters who came to stay with him every once in a while, so I'd rollerblade over there to say hello to my nieces.

One morning, I was at my apartment watching the news. The perky little newslady was talking about a murder or something. I noticed that they were showing my brother's house on the TV! *What?* I got on my bike and rode the five blocks straight over there. *What the fuck? What the fuck? What happened?*

My brother Chris had been caught dealing pot. One of his customers thought he had been shorted on the product or something and went to pay Chris a little visit. Chris thought he heard something outside, so he grabbed his gun and stood on the porch in the dark. (The gun was meant strictly for effect; Chris didn't think it was loaded.)

A figure started moving up the driveway. He was cussing very loud and waving a very large machete. Chris yelled at him to get off the property.

The guy came at Chris and started attacking him. Chris kept trying to use the unloaded gun to pistol-whip the guy, but the gun turned out to be very loaded. It went off and killed the guy.

Someone had called the cops, and they showed up and arrested Chris. He was charged with first-degree murder and use of a firearm in the commission of a murder, but in the end, he was convicted of the lesser charge of manslaughter and the firearms charge instead.

He eventually went to prison, even though it was clearly self-defense. The trial was horrible. The victim's family sat and looked at us like they wanted to kill us.

Chris died in prison at the age of 49.

PART V
REDEMPTION

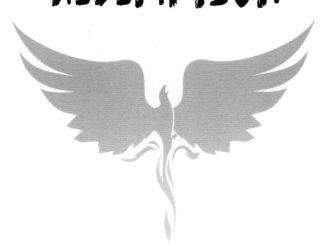

The Bottom, Coming Into View

What they say about improving your life by making a move—a geographical change—well, sometimes it works, sometimes it doesn't.

In 2005, after the long series of mishaps and missteps in Virginia Beach, I landed in Key West. I was back in Dale World, living at his place. He was the only friend I had left. I wasn't legally supposed to be living there, so when the landlord was around, I had to be very quiet or I'd get found out and be kicked off the property.

My days were spent riding my scooter downtown and getting to know the lay of the land, which was really hard. I couldn't figure out how the island was laid out because it didn't go north and south. At that point, my life needed to be simple, but nothing about it was simple—it was hard as fuck. I had no job, and very little money. Dale had a little cash, but he was looking for work, too.

The new Key West M.O. looked like this: Eyes open around nine o'clock in the morning. Some people wake up and light a cigarette; I woke up and did a line of coke, then chugged a half a bottle of wine, mostly to prevent the shakes. That first bump was my version of an espresso double-shot! It elated me and gave me a feeling of comfort and security.

When the liquor store opened in the morning, I'd go in there and get another two bottles of wine and chug one of those before happy hour. Then at night, before I turned off the TV (around 2:30 am), I'd check to make sure I had a line of coke and at least a half-bottle of wine for "breakfast." It didn't have to be chilled; I didn't care. I drank it however it was because I couldn't go without it.

I tried to stop drinking and just do cocaine. Well, that lasted for maybe a day because the cocaine always made me want to drink. And when I did coke, I drank more. But then I'd need more cocaine, which made me need more alcohol to take off the harsh effects of the cocaine. What a vicious, nasty cycle.

OK, so Plan B: Stop doing cocaine and just drink. Well, I would have one martini or two glasses of wine, and then I'd be sleepy and have a blah feeling. Who wants to feel blah? Let's get some drugs. There wasn't a choice to quit one or the other.

I remember one morning talking to Dale before my traditional "breakfast." I had forgotten to set things up for myself the night before, and I was out of both wine and coke. Uh-oh.

He said, "What's wrong with your hands?" I shrugged my shoulders. "Why are they shaking so much?" He actually looked worried.

I could barely lift up a glass. "I don't know. I think I need some alcohol," I said, knowing full well that was exactly why my hands were shaking.

I asked Dale if he had anything around. He gave me the wrong answer, which was "no."

I went and tore up my room, panicking at the thought of no wine at eight o'clock in the morning. I was ripping through my dresser drawers, my closet, my shoes... wherever I might have hidden something. I tore the bed apart. Nothing. I was pleading/yelling at Dale to give me a bump. He kept insisting he didn't have any coke.

Heading back to my room again, I thought I must have had a little bit stashed somewhere. (I always tried to do all that Dale would give me first, and sock mine away for emergencies.) Aha! A little baggie, enough for a line. Now I was jacked, which meant I needed to find some alcohol, but it was too early. (The laws there don't allow alcohol sales until 9:30 a.m.)

Well, I'm kinda cute, right? I'll just go to the liquor store and sweet-talk the guy who works there into selling to me before 9:30. I walked over to the store and grabbed a Smirnoff Ice (because that's not really drinking, it's soda pop, right?) and plunked it on the counter.

"I can't sell you that yet," said the Counter Guy.

Time to turn on the charm. "Please. I'll give you 20 bucks for it."

He was like, "No, I can't." He looked at my hands and saw how bad they were shaking.

"Please, please, let me buy this from you," I whined. He refused again and so I started to go behind the counter. He was trying to size up what the hell I was doing. Was I going to rob him?

"Let me come back there," I purred. "What can I do for you?" I was staring at his crotch, trying to send him the message that I was ready to give him a blowjob. I started undoing his belt.

"Please don't do that," he said. "Stop, stop it. You're embarrassing yourself." He looked at me with a combination of disgust and pity, and handed me back the Smirnoff Ice.

"Just take it and leave," he said. Then he looked at the floor, like he was disgusted with himself as much as he was disgusted with me. I grabbed the bottle and ran out the door. I didn't give a fuck what he thought of me. I got what I came to get.

The second I got outside, I chugged half of it and the shakes went away.

It was hard keeping coke and alcohol around with so little money, so I would often steal it from Dale after he went to sleep. I would wait to hear him start snoring, then I'd pick the lock and very quietly open the door and get some coke out of his bag. Sometimes I'd take the whole bag because I knew that if he'd been partying, he either wouldn't remember what happened to it or he'd think it got lost or fell out of his pocket or something.

By that time, I was truly a bona fide liar, cheat, and thief. Maybe you can even call me somewhat of a whore because I would have done anything for my liquor and my habit. I think I was starting to see the bottom then, but my thinking was so twisted that I could only focus on finding a job to supply all of these addictions.

· 71 ·

FIRED, HIRED AND FRIED

One of the local hotels needed a bartender—yesss! The bar was dark and cool, my kind of place. There were lots of regulars, day-drinkers. I was home.

I loved that job. They let me drink on duty, and that was just amazing. I worked there for about two weeks and got along with everybody because I was a hard worker, and I'd always go above and beyond. It was also scooter-distance from my house. Perfect!

One night after work, I noticed that the manager was hanging around later than he should have. After my shift, he came over and said, "Heather, I need to talk to you." This was serious, whatever it was. I couldn't remember doing anything wrong, but who knows in those days?

I gulped. "What?" He handed me a large, flat manila envelope.

Well, that was scary. I undid the little metal thing and opened it up. It was a picture of me. Not a Glamour Shot... no, it was my mug shot.

I was like, "What is this? How did you get this?" Lots of indignation and stuff. I had no idea that employers could go on the sheriff's website every morning to find out if any of their employees had gotten in trouble overnight, to see who got arrested for what.

It so happens that I had gotten pulled over for driving my scooter the wrong way down a one-way street, along with a long list of other offenses, which I'll talk about in a minute.

"I'm going to have to let you go," he said. I honestly think he didn't want to because at the bottom of everything, I was a good employee.

He explained that if it were just a regular arrest or a DUI, it would be fine, but since there was possession of cocaine in there, I had to go. The Board members were pretty tough on drug use. It didn't matter what he said, though, because I thought I could bargain my way out of it.

"But I wasn't doing it here," I protested.

"Yeah," he said, "but it's on the record and it's public. You're employed here and we don't want people making that connection. We got to let you go."

I was so sad because I really loved that job. To make matters worse, I needed that job. There was only a few hundred bucks to my name and I still had to pay my rent. (I wasn't living with Dale anymore because I had gotten my own room in the same building.)

I'd become good friends with a girl named Cindy, who lived in one of the rooms behind me. She liked to do as much coke as I did. She worked at this restaurant down near the water called Sailor Pete's and she thought she could get me a job there.

So I went for an interview for like my hundredth job. I told them all about my yachtie days and that got them pretty excited.

"Oh, you used to cook? Then you'll be our cook." It was like the last thing I fucking wanted to do. Bartending meant free drinks. Working in the kitchen meant free food, which I didn't care about, but I found a way to sneak a few drinks back there anyway, while I was frying the fish. Pete's manager was pretty hardcore about no drinking at work, so I really had to sneak it. She didn't care about after work, which was great because we'd all sit at the bar and get shitfaced as soon as our shift was over.

Cindy and I often had the same shift, so we would take turns going into the bathroom to tap the little bottle one of us would hide there. I had to have a place to secretly chug my liquor.

Everything had to be preplanned to make sure I had my stuff wherever I was, even if it was in my backpack. People could catch on to that after a while, though, so I didn't haul my backpack to the bathroom a lot. There must have been miniature bottles and coke baggies hidden all over that place, in the potted plants, light fixtures, everywhere. It's amazing someone else didn't find one of my little "hidden treasures." HA!

My perception of things was that I was having fun. This is a good life, I thought. I'm doing what I want. Actually, I was really losing my moral compass.

A guy named Garrett came into Sailor Pete's a lot, and we started hanging out because he was a reliable free coke source. He was pretty nice, so I'd flirt with him, and we'd go to his place and get scary high. One time we rented a room at a cheesy hotel for a night of wild sex, but we got so coked up we didn't even want to be around each other. I couldn't even get a drugged-out derelict to sleep with me! I couldn't see that I was giving him sex for coke. I hate that I did that; I mean I really hate that. It makes me feel so "ick."

My landlord was another piece of work. As long as I paid my rent in cash, he was cool, but if I was late, he'd started pressing me for "interest due." One night he called me and asked me if I'd give him a blowjob. Even I had limits. Not my landlord. Unh-uh.

"Call Cindy and maybe she'll do it," I told him. That's how much respect I had for her.

Work became a drunken comedy of errors. During lunch, I was doing my usual fish-frying thing and a dishrag fell into the fryer. Oh, God, I'm going to ruin the mahi! I instinctively (and stupidly) stuck my hand in the fryer to nab the dishrag. I purposely stuck my hand in the deep-fat fryer. FUCK! MY hand!!

That messed me up for a couple of weeks. I burnt the shit out of my hand and the pain was so intense. Second-degree fryer burns are one of the worst kinds. My coke and alcohol helped ease that some, and my boss let me do some bar-backing instead of cooking so I could still get a paycheck. Lesson learned: Don't drink and fry!

· 72 ·

DOES THIS MAKE ME LOOK FAT?

Now it's time for the mug-shot story. Like I said before, I didn't know my way around Key West very well. There are a lot of one-way streets, which was confusing. One day I put on a cute sun dress and pulled out a cute pocketbook with matching sandals from the back of my closet. I hadn't used that pocketbook for about six months, not since I moved from Virginia Beach. Almost forgot I had it.

Around four o'clock in the afternoon I turned down a one-way street, oblivious to the fact that I was going the wrong way, and motored my little scooter up to the stop sign. About four seconds after I turned right, I heard some blup-blup sirens and a loudspeaker.

"Pull over, pull over," said a deep voice. It scared the shit out of me.

I pulled over. And not one car, not two cars, but three cop cars pulled over with me. You would think I was some kind of international terrorist on a scooter. I did not have a clue what was going on, but I was nervous because at any given time, day or night, I would blow a .30 or higher on a breathalyzer. I was drinking my way around the clock.

The cop slowly swaggered up to me and said, "Do you know why I pulled you over?"

I said, "No, I do not." I was at least telling the truth for a change.

He said, "You just went the wrong way down a one-way street."

My shock was real. "Oh, I didn't know that," I said. "I just moved here about a week ago and I don't know the lay of the land very well."

Then he said, "Can I see your license?"

"No, sir," I said. I wasn't being cheeky or sarcastic, even though the cop thought I was. I really just didn't have a license. That was why I was driving the scooter. You didn't need to have a license in Virginia Beach to drive one. I didn't know what the rules in Key West were, and had never bothered to find out.

So the officer repeated, "I need to see your license."

And I repeated, "Well, I don't have one."

He looked at me pretty seriously and said, "You have to have a license to drive a scooter."

I said, "No, sir, you don't."

He said, "Yes, ma'am, you do."

I said, "Well, in Virginia Beach, you don't. If you have a scooter like this, it's under so many CCs. You don't have to have a license." I suppose that was kind of cheeky, me telling him the law and all.

He sighed and said, "So, do you have an ID?"

And I replied, "No, sir, I don't."

So far, he wasn't getting too pissed off with me. He asked me my name and I told him. He walked back to his car to run my name and see if I had any warrants or anything. He told me to stay where I was.

I had just gotten like my first-ever cell phone, so I flipped it open, called Dale, and told him I thought I was being arrested.

"There are three police cars here," I said. "They said I got to have a license for my scooter."

Dale was like, "Okay, well, you're probably going to be all right," and then just hung up the phone. I only wanted him to be aware of where I was, what the fuck?

The officer came back over to me and informed me that I was driving on a suspended license. Of course, I knew this, which is why I had a scooter, which I thought didn't require a license.

"Yes, sir, again — that's why I'm on this special scooter," I explained, trying to make it seem like I was all law-abiding and stuff.

He got out the handcuffs and said, "Let me see your hands."

"Are you arresting me?" All I could think about was going back to jail again.

He said, "Yes, it's immediate jail when you are driving on a suspended license!" Fuck.

He put me in the back of his squad car, looked at me square in the face and asked, "Am I going to find anything in your scooter seat that you should tell me about?"

"No, sir, just a pair of pink high-top Converses and a bikini," I said, smiling.

He picked up my pocketbook and asked the same thing. God, I hoped there was nothing in there. I hadn't picked up that purse in six months.

He reached all around in there, and when he pulled his hand out, he had a mostly empty baggie of cocaine, with a little left in it.

"I found this in the zipper pouch," said the cop. Shit. I must have forgotten about that.

Then he asked me, "Is this for personal use or distribution?" For real?

So let's add up how much shit trouble I'm in, 10 days after I moved to Key West: Going the wrong way on a one-way street; no license; no registration; driving on a suspended license; and the cherry on top, possession of cocaine. Heather, Heather, Heather.

· 7 3 ·

Do-or-Die Time

We got to the jail, but I wasn't afraid. I remembered the Big Girls from my first time, and how I got up over them and made friends with them. This was going to be another adventure!

The matron did the intake and handed me a black-and-white striped prison uniform, just like in the movies. I was like, "This is so cool that I get to wear this!" Smiling from ear to ear, jumping around like a nut. I'm sure they were thinking this girl was crazy.

Then the adrenalin started wearing off, and all I wanted to do was sleep. Every institution I was ever in, every detox place... it always made me feel new. Finally, I could relax!! It felt like I hadn't slept or really rested for five years.

Two guards led me to a cell without a bunkmate. I immediately went to sleep, and stayed there until they woke me up to eat breakfast. Then I slept some more. Somebody finally came by and told me I could go out to the communal area.

I walked out there and just sat by myself for a bit, taking in what was happening around me. I really just wanted to go back to bed, but they called me and said it was time for my arraignment, so we did a live-video with the judge.

The judge addressed me and said, "You're looking at a felony on your record." As far gone as my brain was, I knew a felony was bad. He said my other option was to do a year in the Drug Court Program, and if I completed it, I would not have a felony on my record. So I opted for Plan B, duh. How hard could it be?

After one night in jail I was released, and Dale called our friend Stan, a taxi-driver friend and another one of my angels. He had picked me up a few times, high, sad, tweaked, you name it. I walked out in the hot sun and there he was.

He looked at me and said, "Heather, you are a beautiful girl. When are you going to stop this crap?" He wasn't giving me a hard time; he was being very kind. I just shook my head and said, "I know."

I was supposed to show up the following Monday to the Drug Court building to submit a urine sample. I could not be positive for any drugs and alcohol, or that was it. Well, I "forgot," and I "dropped dirty," as the saying goes. They sent me to the head of the Drug Court, a tiny little woman named Sandra.

She asked me if I knew why I was in front of her. "Not really," I said.

She sighed and said, "If you have another dirty urine test, I have to put you in jail."

"Oh, okay," I said. "I won't drink, I promise." The alcoholic's famous last words. Just like Dad.

She said, "There's an AA clubhouse around the corner. I suggest you start going to meetings immediately." I really didn't think AA was for me, but I agreed to go. It was better than another stint in jail.

I went to a meeting that night, and it was weird. I heard these people telling stories about drinking, and all I could think of was how much I just wanted a fucking drink! After the meeting, I went to the convenience store and got me a four-pack of Sutter Home wine—small bottles—and downed three of them. What a feeling! Oh wait, shit, I'm not supposed to drink. Oh, well, it was OK, I reasoned, because I had a whole week until my next drug test. I would stop drinking Friday and then I'd be fine to drop a good test on Monday.

Saturday night rolled around, and I found myself having martinis and coke until about 3:00 am. It's OK, I'll get some goldenseal and chug it tomorrow, so I'll pee clean! I thought I knew all the tricks; what I didn't know was that while goldenseal (an herb) can help you pass a drug test, it won't do shit to help you pass an alcohol test.

· 7 4 ·

CALLING ALL ANGELS

Monday came, and because I thought I knew everything, I failed the test and got Strike Two. I was fucking scared. Sandra, the tiny Drug Court judge, called me into her office and she was pissed. I looked at her and started to cry.

"I can't do this, I can't do this," I wailed. "I'm trying not to drink, but I don't have the will power. Can you send me to a detox, please, so I can get a jump-start?"

Very much to my surprise, she agreed. "Let me make a call," she said. I was to go to a detox center about 45 minutes away, and I had to be there at two o'clock the following afternoon. Someone would have to drive me there. Yes, yes, I will go. I was excited!

Dale agreed to drive me. "Look," I said, "Maybe I can get a gram of coke and a bottle of wine, and I can celebrate the whole way there since this is going to be my last time ever drinking or doing cocaine." I was dead serious. Are you kidding me?

To make matters worse, Dale went along with it! We stopped at a liquor store, got the wine (a magnum), and got some coke from the guy on the corner. I just snorted all the coke and chugged all the wine, which is really equivalent to two bottles. By the time I got to the detox place, I was absolutely hammered.

Dale gave me a roll of quarters and said, "I'll see you when you get out. Call me." He was just as clueless as I was.

I knocked on the front door and they buzzed me into this little vestibule area, where they gave me a breathalyzer. The nurse looked like she was going to have a heart attack.

"Oh, my God, we can't let you in." She looked at the breathalyzer again, and shook it, like it might be off or something.

I was like, "Why not?" I knew my tolerance to alcohol and drugs was high, but I could function and didn't think it would show up on their breathalyzer.

My blood alcohol level was .44. A reading of .08 will get you arrested. I was five-and-a-half times over the legal limit, and absolutely should have been dead. A reading of .40 for most people would mean they have fatal alcohol poisoning.

She said, "We can't let you in here because you might have a seizure. You need to go over to detox." I had completely forgotten where I was and didn't understand why this person was talking to me about a hospital. The next thing I knew I was in detox (which was just across the street... how could I have missed that?), with an IV in my arm. I must have been passed out for a long time.

The next thing I remember is sitting in front of somebody at a desk who was asking me all kinds of questions. How much do you drink? How often do you drink? How often do you do drugs? Do your parents do drugs, or did they in the past? Are your parents still alive?

After about an hour of this, I started to feel terrible, really like shit. I couldn't stop shaking. They took me upstairs and they gave me a bed and some Ativan. "Something to relax you," they said. I saw the bed. It was like I had hit the lottery once again. Now I can sleep. Now I can sleep.

The nurses and orderlies were calling me "Earthquake" because I was shaking so violently. They were just trying to get me to eat. They couldn't check my vital signs; I was shaking too bad. After four days in there, I was still shaking. I'd sit in the chair and almost start convulsing. My body was not happy being without the alcohol and the drugs. It wasn't until Day Five that I could actually sort of sit still and eat anything.

My doctor called in a counselor named Caitlin. She was this amazing blind woman who was put on this planet as an angel, I am sure of it. She would talk to me about my drug use, my alcohol, do you know why and how this and that happened, that kind of stuff. She honestly cared.

Things like drawing and painting made me feel calm and good. I started playing cards, and that made me feel somewhat normal. I got the greatest pleasure out of just coloring and doing simple things I'd forgotten even existed: embroidery, sketching, art, you know, little things. It was such a safe, loving space. By Day Nine, I had stopped shaking and I was feeling wonderful.

Before I left the hospital, they filled me with all kinds of good advice. When you leave here, go straight to AA. Get a sponsor and start working the program. You'll be good. If you don't, the chances are slim that you will recover.

All of those kind people, especially Caitlin, had faith in me—and that gave me faith in me, too.

· 75 ·

SLIP AND FALL

Day 10 was the day for me to be released from the hospital. Dale came and picked me up, like he said he would. We were about halfway home and he said we needed to stop for gas. No problem.

Dale got out of the car, and within one second, the addict in me woke up, swooped in and swallowed me whole. That is how fast and evil this disease is, and it is what I hated so much about being an alcoholic drug addict. You just never knew when it was going to hit you and take over. One minute before, I felt awesome and was all ready to start my new, shiny-clean life. One minute later, I was thinking, What's in the ashtray? There's usually coke in Dale's ashtray.

Slowly, I pulled open the tray. It was like a pot of gold at the end of the rainbow. It was saying, Hey, Heather, you can have some. You've been good for 10 days. One bump won't hurt. C'mon, Heather.

A quick look around, and nobody was in sight. I took the keys out of the ignition and put a big old scoop on that key and tooted it. Good, Heather. Now one side feels good. Don't leave the other nostril hanging. Do the other one. Do it.

As soon as I did it, I was like, What the fuck did I just do? I was so ashamed, so mortified, so full of that self-hating "ick" feeling I couldn't stand. I was sobbing, all alone in the car, sobbing and yelling at myself, I can't believe I did that, I can't believe I did that!

Through those raging tears, I saw Dale coming back toward the car and shock set in. I scrambled to tie up the bag and get it back in the ashtray.

He could see that I had been crying. "What's wrong?"

I yelled, "Why didn't you tell me there was cocaine in the ashtray?" As if it was his fault.

"You didn't do it, did you?" he asked. My silence said it all. He didn't come back at me with anything; he just accepted it, like he expected it or something. Well, if Dale wasn't going to hold me accountable, then what's the point?

I said, "Might as well go get me a Smirnoff Ice."

He was like, "Are you sure?" I nodded. Yep, off and running, just like the good old days.

That was Thursday, and I had to report to the Drug Court on Monday, like always. I was freaking out times ten, just freaking out. Now I knew for sure I was going to prison, and that meant my life was basically over. So, what the fuck? Might as well just do the drugs 'cause I'm going to prison anyway.

Leave it to me to come up with a great story for the judge:

Judge, I came back from detox, and went to bed. After I fell asleep, I got up and found a baggie of cocaine in my room, and did it in my sleep, you know, sleepwalking. I didn't realize I had done it 'til I woke up and found that bag on my nightstand.

She'll believe me. I'll be all remorseful and shit. The story had to be believable, but I just went in there and lied my ass off.

"I found this bag on my bed," I lied, and started crying hysterically. "I would never do drugs, never!" My arms were flying around and I was out of control. They were afraid I was going to start hyperventilating, I was crying so hard. Then I realized I was not acting; I really was crying and it wasn't because of going to jail. It was because I was done and my life was over. I might as well just kill myself. That's what I thought. I might as well just kill myself.

After about 20 minutes, they got me settled down and gave me a can of ginger ale.

"Sandra wants to see you," said the bailiff. The news was not going to be good.

I kind of trudged into her office and she looked at me with a real disappointed face. "Heather, I can't believe you," she said. "You were doing so well in detox."

"I know," I replied. "I don't know what happened. I don't. I can't do this. I need a long-term rehab. I can't do this on my own. I can't be out in society. I cannot."

And you know what, that beautiful woman gave me another chance. I could not believe my luck. As I was writing this, I was crying because at that time, there weren't a whole lot of chances left for me.

She said something to me in the sternest voice, looking at me—straight through me—into my soul. I saw empathy on her face, and she said, "Heather, you are killing yourself."

I whispered back, "I know."

When she looked at me, I felt like she could read my sadness and my whole history. I was a wreck, mentally and physically. I weighed 90 pounds.

I told her, "I can't think straight... I need a lobotomy." I was serious. I couldn't not drink because my brain wouldn't allow it. It was controlling me; I wasn't controlling it anymore.

She said, "I will find you something, but you must do exactly as I say. Get your ass home. You don't go to a meeting. You do not come out of your house until I call you. I'm going to find you a bed in a long-term, 90-day rehab. I repeat: You do not come out of your house. Do you hear me?"

"Yes, ma'am. Yes, ma'am. Yes, ma'am." I was so grateful to this kind woman. I would have done anything she said. I was totally on board with this plan. It gave me the structure that I so desperately needed.

· 76 ·

You Can't Turn a Pickle Back into a Cucumber

Judge Sandra called me a day and a half later and said, "I've found a bed for you in a rehab in Miami. You need to be there Thursday and you need to be sober. You do not show up there with ANYTHING in your system." She added, "This is your very, very last chance. I know you can do it. I have faith in you."

I did exactly what she said, and Dale drove me up there, sober as a judge (ha!). That place was a whole new, different atmosphere than the hospital. This was a hardcore, state-funded rehab. There were no tennis courts, no swimming pool. We're talking just the bare necessities.

I checked in with the director and sat there while he looked over my chart. He was like, "Wow, this is quite a record. Are you willing to stay sober and do what you need to do?"

"Yes, sir, I am," I said. I so meant that. I just hoped my brain would allow me to do it.

"All right, then. I'm going to show you your room, which you'll be sharing with three other women."

At my first group meeting, I listened while everyone introduced themselves. They were mostly crack or heroin addicts. I thought, I'm not a crack addict, I'm not a heroin addict, I'm not in as bad a shape as these people. But they scared me, and the director scared me. I didn't like the vibe and I didn't want to be there. I wanted to go home.

No phone calls for the first week, ugh. I felt so alone and brain was so fried that it was hard for me to speak, and even harder for me to retain anything I heard. There was something called "The Acceptance Prayer" that we had to memorize and say every morning. But I couldn't memorize it. I couldn't remember two words strung together. Do this, don't do this, memorize this, say this, not that... it felt like little birds were pecking at me.

The minute I was allowed to make a phone call, it went to Dale.

"Dale, this place is horrible. You need to get me out," I demanded. He said no, so I was stuck there. I know he did it for my own good, but he didn't know what I was dealing with.

One of the counselors was a miserable fuck. He was about 12 years sober, and he was a very bitter man who had decided to take it out on everyone around him. He made it clear that if I broke a rehab rule or did anything wrong that he could send me to jail. Either I marched in step, or went to jail. No gray areas.

That guy used to taunt me, like, "I dare you to break the rules. Give me the pleasure of sending your ass to jail." The guy was always fucking with me.

He decided to make an example out of me early on. He put The Acceptance Prayer on an index card and laminated it.

And acceptance is the answer to all my problems today. When I am disturbed, it is because I find some person, place, thing or situation—some fact of my life—unacceptable to me and I find no serenity until I accept that person, place, thing or situation as being exactly the way it is supposed to be at this moment. Nothing, absolutely nothing, happens in God's world by mistake. Until I could accept my alcoholism, I could not stay sober, unless I accept life completely on life's terms, I cannot be happy. I need to concentrate not so much on what needs to be changed in the world as on what needs to be changed in me and my attitudes.

Then in front of the group, he said, "Okay, this is going to be for Heather. She's going to wear this around her neck until she can recite it, word for word, from memory."

What a motherfucking prick. Aren't these people supposed to be full of love and kindness?

There were other women/girls in there who were breaking the rules, like trying to sneak out. One girl was sneaking around to see her boyfriend, which you were not supposed to do. The idea was to stay away from any possible emotional upset (addiction triggers).

So she ditched rehab, and her guy came and picked her up in his convertible, and they popped a bottle of Champagne in the parking lot. Crazy shit going on there. The whole vibe was so negative. I was trying to keep my head down, trying my best to learn, but I did not want to be there. It was a hot mess.

Sometimes the counselors would take us to a hardcore recovery place on the outside of town called The Little River Club. It was a rough crowd, like Sons of Anarchy, man. But I started listening.

They gave you little perqs for being a good girl. I'd been there a month and they gave me a pass to catch the bus and go to the library. Awesome! I could use the library computer to email Dale, or I could try and call my old best friend, Amy, and tell her I was in rehab. I did that and she was so very, very happy. She has told me since then that when I told her that, she was the happiest she's ever been.

I called my other old friend Alyssa in the Virgin Islands.

"My prayers have been answered," she told me. She was thrilled that I was in rehab and that I was safe. I hadn't had contact with these friends in a long time; they'd all pulled back from me, and they didn't even know the half of how far down I had slid.

But I was doing better. We were doing yoga, and we actually got free medical treatment. I saw a dermatologist, and I got my teeth cleaned, things that normal people do. When you're in the throes of addiction, you don't think about these things.

One month down, two months to go and they upped the ante on the good-girl rewards. Now if I was good, I could get a day pass and catch the Metrorail. I was also allowed to have visitors. Dale came up a couple of times, for my birthday and for Christmas. He wanted to take me to brunch.

Well, that was a real test. There were people drinking mimosas and there was a bar actually in the pool, with people laughing and drinking and having a blast. It made me very uncomfortable. I just wanted to have a nice meal.

Looking back on that, I can see that my will power had gotten a lot stronger and my focus was on the right thing, not the wrong thing. My brain was working a lot better and I realized that Heather was still in there. The good Heather.

· 7 7 ·

BECOMING SOBER: BABY STEPS

After 90 days, it was time to go. Was I ready? Who knows? I was petrified at the thought of being without all of this support around me. I had adjusted to the place and had eventually found some comfort there, but now they had to give my bed to somebody else.

My counselors gave me strict guidelines for what to do when I got home, and that was to go straight to AA, keep going to meetings, and just dive into the AA community. I had to change the people I hung around with, the places I went, the things I did—just like Andy did, remember? I had to divorce myself from my old life, or I would fall right back into drinking and drugging. All of my drug dealers were going to miss my business because I was one of their best customers!

Just before I went to rehab, I told all of my dealers I was going and they were actually happy for me! They bought me chocolates and sodas and all kinds of stuff. I was killing myself and they could see that, and they were so happy I was going to rehab. That strikes me as so funny now.

Without the dealers, that left Dale. My biggest enabler was about to become my biggest cheerleader. He was not going to let me drink or do drugs, and he finally understood that. Now it was time to be fucking serious, because that was the only way I was ever gonna stay sober.

My first trip back to Drug Court after rehab was such a positive experience for me. They were all telling me how great I looked. I sure felt a hell of a lot better. The judge asked me a long list of questions about what I had been doing, if I had been drinking, all that stuff. Because I was still in such a fragile state of sobriety, the judge insisted that I live in a structured environment.

I was not crazy about that idea. I didn't want to live with people anymore. I'd been living with people getting sober, people in every corner of my business for more than three months, and I was really looking forward to living in my own apartment again. I still had my old place; it was all good.

But the court had something else to say about that. They decided I should go and live in a women's shelter for another three months, just to chill and make sure that I had structure in my new sober life. Seeing that I was still in the Drug Court program, I had to comply with all of their rules. And there were a lot of rules.

Off to the women's shelter I went, and it was just like being in rehab except that I could go to work. The staff checked my blood alcohol constantly. I had to meet with a counselor daily. There were group meetings and one-on-one meetings. I had to go to x-number of AA meetings a week. I had a curfew, and chores to do in the shelter. There were a serious number of rules. You know, addicts and alcoholics aren't really good with rules, and I'd had my own rules for a very long time. It was tough to bend like that.

But I had to remind myself that they were just trying to fight for me and get me back to some form of normal. Not brushing your teeth or washing your face for a week is not really how people live. Making your bed, you know, cleaning up after yourself are things you need to do. Oh, yeah. I should take a shower. I actually would forget to do that. Those are the most basic things I had to re-learn. I had to learn to live in civil society all over again because of all the years of drugs and alcohol, all the years I lived in Heather-Netherworld. I counted it up one day and realized I had spent nearly two-thirds of my life in the grip of that shit.

First on the agenda was to get a job, because I had to pay rent to the shelter. The AA people constantly tell you that you should stay away from people, places, and things that are triggers from your old life, so finding a job was hard. All I knew how to do was cook and bartend. Well, bartending was out, and cooking, well my yacht-chef days seemed so far removed. Knowing me, finding another job on a boat would have been a huge trigger and a huge mistake anyway. What the hell was I going to do?

Then I saw an ad in the paper for an assistant dock master at a marina. I figured, well, I'd worked on a boat. I know how to tie up lines on the dock and stuff like that. It would be my first test of how well I could cope with real life. I went for it and I got it. Baby steps!

· 78 ·

BECOMING SOBER: THE "ICK"

I was four months sober. I had put down all the substances, even pot. Life without booze and drugs is still really odd, to this day. Drinking was almost like an appendage for so long; giving it up was like losing a best friend, or a lover. You're like, What do I do with myself now? You're sort of like in a state of grief. It is a loss, after all—you don't have it anymore. But you go on if you want to live.

The challenge in front of me was not only how to live without substances but even more about how to live with myself and confront the deep, deep shame—the "ick" I've mentioned—I felt when I thought about the things I'd done and said. Basically, I had no self-confidence or self-esteem.

I was still the phoenix that hadn't yet risen from the ashes. I had crashed and burned and now I had to learn to walk again. I was so nervous about almost everything I did, just scared of my own shadow.

I mustered up what little courage I had, went down to the marina, and asked for an application. There was a really nice girl named Sheila there. She said, "Well, it'll be nice to have another girl here." I guess she liked me.

The application had a space for computer experience. "I've never worked on a computer before," I admitted. I felt like an antique. This was 2006.

"Don't worry," said Sheila. "We'll teach you that. Let us run your application by the general manager, and we'll let you know."

They called me a couple of days later and told me to come down and start to train. I was riding a bicycle, because I still had no driver's license. I was honest with them and told them that I had a really strict schedule where I was living, and I had to be in by ten o'clock every evening. One of their shifts was 2:30 to 10:30, but the shelter wound up bending that rule for me so I could get that job.

Before I got hired, I had to meet the general manager, Mason. I went into his office, and the first thing he said was, "So, you're newly sober?"

"Yes, sir, I'm four months sober." I swallowed hard, hoping I hadn't just lost this job opportunity.

He said, "Well, I know how hard it is to get sober because I'm twelve years now."

What a relief! This is so nice. I will have a real ally who gets it!

The man was so generous to say, "You know, if at any time you're feeling like you have to drink and you need to hit a meeting, just let me know and we'll let you go." I thought that was one of the kindest things I had ever heard. It was pretty, pretty cool.

They patiently trained me, and the job was going well. Everything was hard for me because I felt like I really didn't have the capacity to learn anymore. I didn't retain stuff very well because I had destroyed so many brain cells with all that alcohol. Slowly but surely, though, I made my way and I enjoyed working there.

A couple of times it was suggested to me that I might want to work in the clubhouse kitchen, knowing that I had all that cooking experience. Honestly, I didn't even want to cook when I moved to Key West. I was so fried, so burned out. (There are enough puns for a whole year.)

It took me about two years to even turn on a stove in my own house because it brought back so many memories of Pegasus and all the other bars and restaurants and boats I'd worked on (and been fired from). All things associated with those days would make me feel that "ick" shame, remorse, and just how very, very gross I was.

After a while, I discovered that if I said I didn't know what to do, people would suggest things and help me out. That was great because it let me put myself in the hands of people I trusted. I couldn't trust myself. I still didn't know what was good for me or bad for me.

At the six-month mark, someone at work told me they needed a counter person at the clubhouse. "We think you should do that," they said, and fear shot through me like a bullet. Oh my God, that means I'm going to have to talk to people. I'd have to interact with customers, and I might even need to hold my head up and look people in the eye. So scary.

My bosses were honest and upfront, and they guaranteed it would be scary, but it was necessary for me to grow and help me stay sober. I'd told them I'd do anything to stay sober, so I took the counter job. They were very supportive and I'll never forget them for that.

Serving coffee, sodas, and such was fine, but I'd have to say, "Hello, how are you?" I would just give them just a darting glance and then put my head back down. Oh, my God. I just tried to repeat over and over that this was helping my sobriety.

I found a sponsor, who is kind of like a cross between a mentor, a friend ,and a hall monitor. It was another pillar in my support system. The guy asked me, just like the judge, "Are you willing to go to any lengths to stay sober?" At that point, I absolutely, absolutely was.

· 79 ·

BECOMING SOBER: PROGRESS, NOT PERFECTION

Life was starting to have a routine, a rhythm. I was learning how to live with myself without drinking and how to deal with everyday problems without cocaine or alcohol to help me feel better. I was pretty damn fortunate. About five months into sobriety, I woke up one day and realized I wasn't thinking about alcohol. That, to me, was a huge win-win day!

A new phase of Drug Court began, and I had to go in front of a new judge once a month to report on my progress and what was happening in my life. If I messed up, I'd go to jail.

The very first time I went to Drug Court I had a nice dress on because my mom always said, "When you fly, when you go to church, when you go to court, you always need to look nice." And so I dressed appropriately. I was always pretty astounded at how so many people were dressed in court. How are they going to please the judge looking like that? Maybe that's just the way some people were brought up, but not me.

It was petrifying to stand in front of the judge and a hundred and fifty other people and say anything, let alone talk about myself. One of my counselors was with me, so that helped some. The judge asked me a couple of questions, and I just answered yes sir, no sir.

Then the judge looked at the whole courtroom and said, "You all look at this young woman right here." Oh, he was going to tell all the people how well I was doing. What a nice man.

He continued. "I want you guys to see this girl. She's going to be one of the ones to fail. She's not going to pass this program, I guarantee it."

I couldn't believe it. He had the balls to say that in front of the whole court. I was so pissed off, but I didn't talk back. Why would he say that? I was starting to choke back tears and mumbled something obscene under my breath.

He jerked his head around and snapped at me. "What did you say?" He thought I was disrespecting him.

I said, "Nothing, your Honor, I was clearing my throat." I turned to my counselor, trying to keep it together. I couldn't understand this attitude of his, and still don't. It was my first time in front of that guy. But I had to go to Drug Court, so each month, I went in and gave it my 100%.

The whole point of this program was to find out what that gaping hole in my soul was all about. Why was there such a big hole and why was I using drugs and alcohol to try and fill it? What could I do to feel better about myself, to feel like I deserved to be on this planet, without drugs and alcohol? For most of my life, I didn't care. I wasn't really engaged in life and I didn't have a whole lot to live for. When I drank and did drugs, I thought I felt better, but what I was really doing was committing suicide on the installment plan.

Learning how to get honest with myself was one of the hardest things. We all think honesty means not telling a lie to other people, but honesty is also not telling a lie to yourself. It means learning to live with the shit that's inside you.

I went to seven AA meetings or more a week, and did a lot of work with my sponsor. I had always heard that AA was a cult, and I was never going to be in a cult, but then I started to notice that I was an awful lot like these other people who I once thought were nothing at all like me.

It's funny because in AA, people are always walking around quoting things and sayings all the time. In the beginning I would think, Oh, my God, I could never sound like these people. I will never talk like that.

Well, now I kind of talk like that a little, Haha! But it's not a cult; it's a way of changing the way you think and dealing with your problems head-on. In the past, I'd just bury my problems in alcohol and cocaine. When I finally came out of that haze, the problems were still there. To be a responsible, sober adult, I had to learn how to deal with them.

The more sober I got, the more comfortable I got in my own skin. Still, it was hard. I still didn't feel pretty or worthy. I still felt like no guy thought I was attractive. It's hard to stop that tape from looping in your head, over and over and over again.

The "ick" that I hated so much... how was I going to get rid of the "ick" feeling? That was the question of the day. I still get the "ick," but now I understand that it is shame. Shame and disgust at the things I said, the things I did, the people I hurt. The power to cope with that was something I had to reach outside of myself for, you know, find a higher power to help me handle it.

People wonder what a "higher power" is. I would describe it as something in the universe that is bigger and more powerful than yourself. You can call it whatever you want: God, Buddha, Allah, whatever.

That concept was hard for me because I'm a visual person. I need to see what I'm praying to and talking to. I want to make sure I'm going to get some answers. Well, it doesn't work that way, and that's why they call it "faith."

Maybe above everything, I really needed not to be judged. I needed love, loyalty, and even humor to be inside of me. I used to always love to laugh; it made me feel alive. So I started praying and asking for all these things. The main thing was, of course, "Please don't let me drink today. Please don't let me drink today." The more I prayed, the farther and farther away drinking drifted from my thoughts.

· 80 ·

BECOMING SOBER: WORKING THE PROGRAM

Every once in a while, like riding back home from work, I would stop at a corner and feel how hot the sun was. Wow, a nice cold gin and tonic at the Jiggernaut would be so awesome right now! Well, number one, I'd never hung out at the Jiggernaut and number two, I never drank gin! So that is how your brain starts to fuck with you a little bit. Well, just one won't hurt. Just one won't hurt. It's that devil on your shoulder.

To get past those moments, I learned to think about how far I had come, and how I felt the last time I drank. Was it an image of an ice-cold martini, listening to music on the balcony of a swanky hotel? Well, fuck no. It was drinking warm bottles of cheap-ass wine, sleeping on a dirty floor. And if I couldn't get the bottle open, I'd smash the top and drink out of the jagged glass. That's how it was the last time I drank. Does that appeal to me? Fuck no.

Sometimes I would get a fleeting thought of walking down to the docks at sunset, when people are having Champagne with all those pretty beads of condensation on the cold bottle. The waiter would pour it into those pretty glasses with those elegant little bubbles. The thought is like a beautiful TV commercial.

Maybe just one glass, Heather? And then my program kicks in. When was the last time you had a nice glass of Champagne, Heather? Well, you never had one glass. The last time you had it, you probably drank some cheap California shit and then went to the drug man. There's never a good ending to that thought.

It's really about keeping myself in the present on a moment-to-moment basis. I don't think about the future, except as a series of guideposts. My sponsor asked me to write down five goals that I wanted to complete in the next five years. When I was seven months sober, I wrote this list:

1. I would like to have a driver's license.
2. I would like to have a bank account.
3. I would like to have my own place to live.
4. I would like to have some friends.
5. And I would like to have my family back in my life.

Do you have all those things? Most people have had these things for a very, very long time. But remember, I was starting over. I hadn't had any of these things in forever because I was living the life of a drug addict and an alcoholic. I thought these things were so far-fetched that I wasn't ever going to be able to accomplish them. But I wrote them down anyway.

A few months more into my counter job at the clubhouse, a woman walked in. I looked up at her and asked, "Hey, how are you doing?" I really wanted to know.

"Fine," she said. I asked her name and actually started a conversation. I felt like a butterfly, just coming out of the chrysalis and opening my wings, that phoenix finally rising from the ashes. I was beginning to lift my head up and become a real person again.

I worked that job for about a year, and then started washing boats on the side. After four months or so, they let me out of the shelter. I still had to go to Drug Court and report in once a month, but I was so happy to go back to my little 10 x 10 room I had before I went into rehab.

I was even happier to find that my awesome neighbor had cleaned out my room while I was gone. When I left, it had empty wine bottles all over the floor, empty cocaine bags that had been licked clean, and licked again. It looked like a shithole, like a crack den. But when I came back, it was so clean and nice. I was so grateful for that.

Gratitude is a big part of the program. There are 12 steps in all and you have to work them. I was doing that, living the steps. Step 3 is to trust your higher power and not react to things. Like when somebody cuts you off in traffic, your first thought should not be to honk and flip them off. So then what if somebody is driving super-slow right in front of you, and you've got somewhere to be? Well, I take myself out of the equation and play a little game with myself. I "levitate" above the situation, look down, and I make a story up.

This car is going so slow because it's a cute old tourist couple who don't know the area and they're looking for the southernmost point on the island. They've got their maps out because they don't know how to use a GPS. They're really admiring the palm trees and the beautiful, beautiful island I get to live on.

The alternative is for me to behave like a screaming howler monkey, honking and yelling and wondering why the fuck they're not going at my pace. If I can take myself out of the equation and be more selfless, then I can keep myself pretty much drama-free.

That takes a lot of practice, you know. If somebody suddenly comes up to me and they're angry and shouting at me and I have no idea why, then I ask myself, Is my side of the street clean?

If I haven't done anything to this person, then my side of the street is clean. So the question becomes, Why are they projecting their anger onto me? It's not about me at all. It's about them and their fear and their insecurities and their shit. It's such a relief to learn to think that way.

Another thing I had to practice was patience. I would purposely go to the Winn-Dixie at five o'clock in the afternoon—the busiest time—and choose the longest checkout line and let the person behind me go in front of me. That's how we practice patience and tolerance.

Bonus points: When I get to the cashier and he is being snippy because he's having a rough day, I smile and ask him how his day is going. His whole demeanor will change.

Another little trick I do to make myself to feel better is this: If I see somebody having a cruddy day and they're just in their own shit (this frequently happen to anyone who serves the public, especially in retail), I will find something to compliment them on, like, "That's a really pretty blouse that you have on," or, "I love your shoes." "Really?" they'll say, and just brighten right up. When you practice that, you get people out of their own shit. You'd be amazed at how you can make people's day when you just do those random acts of kindness. Just open your mind and get out of your own fucking way. That's what I say.

At about the nine-month mark, I went to the Virgin Islands to visit my old and dear friend, Alyssa. The last time I saw her was a few years earlier on a visit. My alcoholism was in full swing then. I was hiding bottles in fast-food bags, sneaking them in the house, and hiding them in the toilets, under my bed, and in my pillowcase.

One afternoon, we went to a PTA meeting at her son's school. Alyssa had volunteered to set up for some big party, and I offered to come along and help. Of course, I had vodka in my orange soda can, but she didn't know that. She had no idea how much I'd really been drinking.

The party started rolling, and I was having fun with my vodka and orange soda. Next thing you know, I was getting loud and embarrassing. I remember Alyssa grabbed my arm and pulled me into like an adult time-out.

"You sit right here and don't say another word," she said. She was super-pissed.

"But I need to go get another drink," I said. "I'm all out."

"Heather, there's no alcohol here. What is WRONG with you?" She was so upset at me. Then she looked at the soda can. "Do you have vodka in there?"

Well, hell yeah, I had thought it was supposed to be a party. She just shook her head in disgust. To this day, I'll never, ever forget that. She and I can joke about it now, thank God.

It was so good to see Alyssa again a few years after that and enjoy her company without constantly looking in every corner for some alcohol. It was important, however, even though I was technically on vacation, to go to AA meetings. I found a local chapter that met in the basement of a church, and Alyssa took me there. Not a lot of confidence yet, and my footing wasn't very solid, but I went.

I walked up to the church and thought I would ask the guy at the top of the stairs to point me to the meeting spot. As I got closer, I could clearly see that I knew this person.

It was my old boyfriend, Andy, the Mel Gibson lookalike and crack addict. Andy. The last time I saw him he told me he couldn't see me anymore because he had gotten sober and couldn't be around all of my drinking and drugs. One of my heartbreakers.

Well, he was probably about seven years sober by that time. He was genuinely glad to see me and gave me a big hug. I was in a mild state of shock. He looked great, so healthy. We went inside to the meeting and he introduced me to everyone.

You may or may not know that at an AA meeting you're invited to tell "your story."

Well, Andy played a huge part in my story, so the situation was kind of awkward. It was my turn and I stood up.

I look at him and mouthed, "I'm sorry," and then I told my tale. At the same time, the other half of my brain was thinking, He looks pretty hot. Hmm… maybe we should reignite that fire? It's so hysterical the way my brain works. I was there for one thing, but I always had another motive, you know? It was nice, though, because he and I were on a sober-wavelength friendship. And guess what? We're still Facebook friends today. He's happily married and is living his life to the fullest. I'm really thrilled for him.

And so nine months of sobriety turned into one year, a very big deal. I was kind of bummed out because everybody in AA celebrates 30 days, six months, nine months, and then a year. But then what? They're not going to celebrate me anymore until I get a whole 'nother year under my belt.

What's that talking there? Ego, right? That's selfishness, right there. I nearly sabotaged myself by thinking that way. Maybe if I don't make it a year, I can start all over with my 30 days, 60 days, etc. I'll get all the applause and attention again. Yay!

That is faulty thinking, and the fact that I know it's faulty thinking means I've been working on my inner growth instead of looking for the accolades of "YAY"— but understanding that at the same time, applause and attention can be rewarding and reassuring. Whenever I had those faulty thoughts, I would tell them to someone else in the program, or to my sponsor. I didn't hide things from people anymore. No secrets.

It was really good in my early years because I would call my sponsor and start ranting about crazy shit that made no sense (although it made perfect sense to me at the time).

And then he would just calmly say, "Well, did you pray today?"

Of course, I'd say something rude like, "What the fuck does praying have to do with this?"

"Did you pray today?"

I was like, "No!"

He'd say, "Why don't you try and pray? We'll have this conversation later."

What the fuck? So I prayed, and then whatever crazy shit was in my mind would go away. We call that "move a muscle, change a thought." Do something physically different and you will think differently. It works.

Those are just some of the little tricks I had to learn in order to live with myself and to not want to pick up a drink.

Along the way I have also discovered that the people I thought were my friends were really nothing more than just drinking and drug-buddies. When I got sober and quit hanging out at the bars, my whole group of "friends" became non-existent because we no longer had anything in common.

I began to wonder if I was ever going to have any real friends in my life. For the longest time I thought everything was going to simply revolve around going to work and cleaning boats.

· 8 1 ·

TOE IN THE WATER

My sober life was taking off. I was finally meeting some friends—not a lot, but I was at least meeting new people. Much of my free time was spent hanging out with my AA peeps, which I actually found to be a lot of fun. We'd go out to dinner and laugh so loud that we'd be asked to leave... no alcohol involved. The irony!

My sense of humor used to be pretty legendary (all fueled by alcohol, of course). But now I had to find out if my real personality had a good sense of humor as well. I felt like I had 14 thumbs and no fingers, just fumbling around in the dark, trying to make shit work. It wasn't always easy. Not always easy, but a whole hell of a lot better.

I started to think about dating again. They always say to stay away from emotional situations during your first year; don't get involved in romantic relationships or dating sites or booty calls. All that lusting takes away the sunlight from your spirit.

But we all know that a first kiss can set you on fire, especially if there's good chemistry. Then all you can do is think about that guy... think about that guy... think about that guy. And here's the thing—if I'm constantly just thinking about that guy, I'm not thinking about staying sober. More faulty thinking.

I know that, and I started getting away from what I had been learning about myself, and what not to settle for. After so many years of looking in the mirror and not being able to stand what I saw, I was starting to feel pretty okay about the way I looked. Before, it was like an old witch looking back at me, and that was sad. But now? I can raise my head a little bit and have a little confidence.

When I first hit a year of sobriety, I decided to go on one of those dating sites, just dip my toe in. As I was scrolling through the profiles, I had my sights set on an awesome, ideal guy. But you know what they always say: Be careful what you wish for.

I found this one guy that I planned to meet. Before our "date," I must have changed my clothes 40 times. The thing I worked hard to remember was that this was just a date, not a marriage proposal. No rush. No pressure. No wham, bam, we're getting married, which never happened for this girl, ha!

So Mr. e-Date was about four-foot eight. Really short. He didn't look short in his picture. We did have some things in common, so why not? The one thing I didn't realize about him was that he drank. We went to one of those movie theaters that serves drinks, so we ordered something and sat through the movie.

I was so insecure and self-conscious and uncomfortable! I did not enjoy myself at all. He was like, "Well, how about we go grab some dinner?" This was about 8:30. I was like, "No, I got to go home." He said, "Well, we could..." and I was still like, "Nope, I got to go home."

So I ran like a scared dog with its tail between its legs. It took way too much out of me. I guess I wasn't what we would call "spiritually fit" yet. And with no alcohol to lubricate me, it was extra-hard. When you're still figuring out who you are and what your personality really is, it's hard to go one-on-one with a stranger.

On the second try, I had a little better luck. I tried a site just for people who are into fitness and landed on this guy named Geoff. We talked for a couple of months, but didn't meet right away. He lived up north but also had a winter house in Florida. He was supremely hot. Six-feet-four inches, blue eyes, retired military, built like a shit-brick house. Handsome, and funny. And he had a sailboat. Oh, my God, those beautiful blue eyes. We know what blue eyes are about! More about him later.

In the midst of my third year, I found out that Dale (from the Pegasus days) had passed away. He was only 54. All that coke wrecked up his heart and I think the restaurant closing was harder on him than anyone knew. I never had the chance to make amends with him, and that is something I'll always regret.

In 2009, my four-year anniversary was coming around, and I was feeling really good. I'd gotten my best friend, Amy, back in my life, as well as my sister Elizabeth. My brother and sister-in-law, my niece and nephew, they were all back in my life, too.

One of the steps in my recovery meant I had to make amends about the crap and actions that I did to other people. Not like, just go up and say, "I'm sorry" because I had said "I'm sorry" a lot.

When I was drinking and drugging, "I'm sorry" really meant "get me out of my shit." Get me out of trouble. It wasn't like I really was sorry that I hurt your feelings. I was sorry that I made you worry over me all these years.

That's what I found out when I was making my amends with these people— they weren't being mean to me by pulling themselves away from me. They were just protecting their hearts. I didn't know that because I was in my own shit. It was all about me, you know.

They were all very worried, and they couldn't watch me kill myself. They couldn't watch me being in an emotionally abusive, trapped relationship where I was being controlled by men and alcohol. They couldn't stand looking at how sad I was all the time. That was breaking their heart and they knew they couldn't do anything about it. For them, it was like watching somebody who you absolutely love, self-destruct.

I made my amends to the people that I needed to. I know it's going to take the rest of my life because I don't remember everybody or every thing I did. From time to time I will remember, and I'm like, shit. I'll remember I did this, or I did that to that person. But as long as I keep honest and I keep sober, it'll be all right.

In my second year of sobriety, someone at a meeting told me about a "boot camp" aimed at getting you in great physical shape. It was on the Boca Chica Navy base. An amazing man, Retired Master Chief Tommy Taylor, ran it for free. He was all about bettering yourself, both mentally and physically. I had no confidence and I hadn't worked out in years, so I was nervous about going.

I remember showing up in the pitch-black early morning (5:30) by myself. A nice girl, Debbie, introduced herself and I met a bunch of other amazing athletes. I was not on their level at all! We would run and do all kind of stops, run fast, stop, do burpees, pushups, pullups, and I had to work very hard to keep up.

That's when I found out I had asthma. I would get to the point where I had exercise-induced asthma, and Tommy would slow me down, run with me, and get me relaxed. He had the most amazing way with people. He wanted us all to push ourselves to our greatest potential and that man gave me confidence and self-esteem. I give a lot of credit for my success to Tommy! I would do anything this man asked me to do; I owe him a lot. Our group is called "The PT Raiders." My tribe, my people.

We addicts and alcoholics often exchange one obsession for another—and of course, mine was working out and getting the fittest I could ever be. There's never a middle ground for me; it's all or nothing.

—◇○◇—

PART VI
CANCER

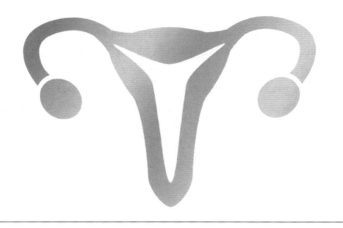

Cancer, Schmancer

Four years passed and I was really working/living my program. I felt so happy! I got a bank account. I got my license back. I'd actually traveled a bit and went to see my brother. Amazingly, I was still washing boats and making money *at the same job*. I was making real progress on that five-year Sober Bucket List!

When I was first sober, I got a personal trainer (Courtney) at the gym and decided I was going to sign up for a fitness competition. My health became a serious priority for me. I changed up my diet, was getting my eight hours' sleep, and was training hard, all while working at the marina and washing boats on the side. For the first time in a long time, I felt really good because I was in great shape. It was strange, though, because I felt tired all the time. Then I noticed I was gaining a little weight in my belly, maybe over the course of two weeks or so. It didn't make any sense.

"Courtney, fuck, we're working a lot of core," I complained. "I think you're building my abs backwards because my lower abs are starting to pooch out." I was pretty annoyed, considering all the hard work I was doing. "You need to change this shit up *now*."

"What are you eating?" he asked, puzzled. I said I was on my strict eating program, doing everything I was supposed to do. (I was *perturbed*, but not angry. I quit doing that emotion. It takes a lot to push me to the edge... I mean, a lot.)

Courtney was mystified. He said he hadn't changed anything in the workout routine. Then I remembered that it was time for my period, which was usually very light. That time, it was very heavy. *Was that it?*

A checkup was probably a good idea, so I went to one of the local clinics. They did an ultrasound and a sonogram. The loopy doctor—who seemed like she was drunk (Ha! One of me, drinking on the job)—came in and told me I had a fibroid tumor on my uterus.

I said, "Well, can you please schedule surgery to take it out?" Thank God, I had really good insurance at the marina.

She just shook her head and explained that fibroid surgery was considered "cosmetic" and that insurance wouldn't cover it.

I was like, "What do you mean, 'cosmetic surgery'? You just told me I had a tumor?"

She said, "Yeah, but fibroid tumors are generally benign and it'll go away when you hit menopause. Fibroids are very common."

My jaw dropped. I was too fucking young to hit menopause. You mean I have to walk around with this fucking spare tire around my waist until I hit menopause? *You have got to be fucking kidding.*

I was devastated. *Devastated.* My body image was a big deal to me and that was just not the way I rolled.

I didn't tell very many people about it. I always have been very independent, wanting to work things out on my own and not be a bother. Why trouble other people when I can figure it out myself? That attitude is probably what got me in trouble in the first place.

There was a holistic doctor in town, so I made a plan to go see her and maybe she could just "acupuncture it out." That was funny, especially when you said it out loud to a doctor. Oh, my God, I crack myself up sometimes.

But she humored me and she did it. Unfortunately, the spare tire remained, and now I was really sad *and* depressed *and* tired all the time. This thing was sucking all my red-blood energy cells or something. I was trying to do the very physical job of washing boats, but It was taking me twice as long as it used to. I just had no strength or energy.

Somebody told me about an awesome gynecologist in town. What the hell? I said I'd give it a shot because I didn't have a better idea, and I couldn't go on that way because it was really stressing me out.

(You might wonder if a stressful thing like that made me want to drink. That's when your brain has to go to work. I could have just said, *Fuck it, get a goddamn drink. They can't help me, so fuck it.* Nope, never. Ain't gonna happen. I just accepted the fact that I was going to be fat the rest of my life. Even former bulimics don't like the thought of being fat, but if that's the deal, that's the deal. But I am not going to drink because of it.)

The gynecologist had the most amazing energy, and she was so kind. She asked me what was going on. I immediately started crying and explained everything in a lot of short, sniffly sentences. She got that this thing was really upsetting to me.

"I tell you what we're going to do," she said. "We're going to watch this for a month. After a month, if it's still the same, we will take it out. If it *grows* by the end of the month, then we're going to have to figure something else out because maybe it's not just a fibroid tumor."

I was like, okay, because I'm not one to go straight to the negative or jump on the computer and get a bunch of scary (and wrong) information from Google. That's not me. So I waited.

As the month went by, I was getting more tired and more tired, and fatter and fatter. My stomach was just growing, like, *man, there's something wrong.* I wasn't even worried that something bad might have been inside me. My main thing was that I was getting fatter. And people were going to think I was fat. *That was horrible.*

At the beginning of the month, the tumor was four centimeters. At the end of the month, it was 16.5 centimeters.

"Oh, my God! You look four months pregnant," said the doc. I was like, *Fuck me.* "Look, I think it's something more, but I don't know for sure. I'm going to send you to a gynecologist friend of mine up in Boca. He's really hot." She winked at me. "Here, I'll make you an appointment for next week. Okay?" *Sure, okay.*

After another week of tiredness and fatness, I went up to Boca (by myself) for the consultation. It wasn't much of a big deal to me and I didn't feel the need to call in the cavalry just yet. It wasn't like it was a brain tumor or something.

I waited in Dr. H's office while he saw another patient. (I called him "Dr. H" for "Doctor Hot.") His office was gorgeous (so was he), all dark wood. He had a model of a longhorn on his desk and I wondered if he was from Texas. *Who knows.*

When he came back in, he said, "Heather, I think we got a little bit more going on than just this fibroid." For the first time, the C-word popped into my head. It had never come my way: no family, no friends... I never knew anybody who had cancer. *Cancer, schmancer,* just like Fran Drescher said.

"I want to schedule an immediate hysterectomy," he said. He was serious. After that little announcement, he launched into a bunch of technical stuff. I didn't understand a fucking thing he said. My eyes just glazed over and he could tell I wasn't getting it.

Dr. H. got up, came around the desk, and sat right next to me. I thought he was going to draw a picture on his pad of paper.

He pointed to the model of the "longhorn" and said, "So this is your uterus."

Oh my fucking God, oh Lord, oh, my God! How stupid am I? I thought it was a longhorn steer.

I started cracking up and he looked at me like I was a fucking lost cause. Hysterical.

So he drew his picture and said something about eggs and stuff. I didn't get any of it but I said okay and he told me to schedule the surgery at the reception desk out front.

I'm not sure how I got home; I was kind of on auto-pilot. The first thing I did was call my sponsor and told him I had to have a hysterectomy. He was sympathetic and agreed to drive me up to Boca when the time came. Maybe it was time to tell my sister?

· 83 ·

Laughter Is Not the Best Medicine—Morphine Is

I was still talking to Geoff from the fitness-dating site (we still hadn't met yet), but I wasn't going to tell him anything about the hysterectomy because it wasn't a big deal. I was even asking my friends and my sponsor how long I had to wait to have sex after a hysterectomy. Too funny, but I really wanted to know because I was planning to meet him in a month or so. Everyone was just laughing at me.

The next day I was scheduled for the surgery, which fell on the same day as my four-years-sober anniversary. I checked in, filled out tons (and tons) of paperwork and waited (and waited). After what seemed like forever, they got me into the operating room.

I wasn't nervous; I was excited that I was going to get a "legal high." *I'm going to get some drugs because they're going to put me under.* This was a freebie for me!

The anesthesiologist joked, "Would you like a margarita before we get started?" My fleeting thought was like *Hey, nobody will know,* but I told him, "I can't."

"Well, I'll give you one anyway," he said as he started the anesthetic drip. He told me to count backwards, and I was out. I woke up in my hospital room.

When I opened my eyes, my sponsor was there. I was in so much pain. I felt like somebody was stabbing me like a voodoo doll. I started crying because the pain was so bad. *So* bad.

My sponsor buzzed for the nurse, and in a minute this guy came in. "What is the problem here?" he said. Really snarky.

"You need to give her something," said my sponsor. The nurse said that I wasn't scheduled to have anything, which made both of us mad.

The nurse seemed almost happy to say, "Well, you know, she's just going to feel worse before she gets better!" *Are you serious?*

My sponsor and I said almost at the same time, "Give her some damn pain medication!" I guess the nurse realized it really was necessary, and he hooked me up to some morphine. *Mmmmm.*

Best drug I ever did in my life. Every time I was in pain, I yelled, "Push the button, push the button!" And my sponsor would push the button, push the button.

"By the way, do you know what day it is?" he asked. I was like, "No," because I really didn't. "Happy fourth-year anniversary, baby!" Yep, it was my four-year sober anniversary and I was all doped up on morphine. How's that for messed up?!

The entire thing was like the old game "Operation" to me. I didn't know what the doctors had done (I do now). I thought they just went in and picked stuff out without touching the sides, and then, you know, game's over and you go home.

The doc came in to see me the next day. "I took your ovaries and I took your uterus," which was kind of a shock to me, but I started laughing to myself anyway. Oh good, did that mean I would lose some weight? HA!

"You mean you took out the longhorn?" I said, laughing. I could make a joke out of anything. The worse the situation, the funnier I got. They say you need three bones to get through life: A wishbone, a backbone and a funny bone. So true.

He said, "We saw something, maybe on your ovary, but I think you're going to be fine. As of right now, you're good."

I was like, "Awesome. When can I go home?"

"Well, you've got to poop before you can go home." *Did he really say I had to poop?*

It was the next day and I still hadn't pooped or farted. Finally, that afternoon, I passed a big-ass fart. My niece, who was up at the hospital with my sister, started jumping up and down and running down the hallway.

"Heather Feather farted, Heather Feather farted!" She was yelling at the top of her lungs and then ran right into my sponsor. He was like, "Why are you so excited?"

"Heather Feather farted," she yelled. She was excited because she knew that meant I could go home.

After that momentous event, the doctor came back. "Look, I had to cut your ab muscle a little bit. You probably won't have the abs that you had before." *What bullshit is that? I'm not listening to that.*

He added, "But the scars are below your bikini line." Well, thank God for small favors. My ego felt a little better. Then he said, "You can't work out for a long time. You can't lift anything more than three pounds. If you do, your bladder could fall out."

I stopped dead in my tracks. "Excuse me?"

"Yeah, your bladder could fall out."

I was trying to think about where the fuck my bladder could fall out of. I looked down and pointed to my vagina.

"Yes," he said. *Holy fuck!*

Then he explained that everything had to be cut to get to the bad stuff and get it out. After that, he basically stuffed everything back in and sewed it up to hold it in place, so things were just a little wobbly in there. Well, he did what he had to do.

· 84 ·

Humans Make Plans... God Laughs

I was finally discharged and went home. I couldn't work for a month. Thank God x10 for my good insurance.

After being home for about a week, I was thinking I was in the clear. The doc took an awful lot of stuff out of there, so he must have gotten any bad stuff along with it. Then I got a call from the doctor, who had said he would follow up with me.

"Heather, I need to see you in my office on Tuesday." What is up with this? I thought I was done with this.

"I'd much rather tell you here that we might have found something."

Oh, what now? "I thought you got everything?" I had things to do, places to go, etc.

"Yeah. I'd just like to discuss it with you up in here the office," he said. I rented a car and drove up there. This whole thing was getting kind of dark.

The doctor explained that when the pathologist looked at the ovaries, he thought there might have been a cell there, but it was only half a cell. "We're going to send it over to the Yale Institute, because this is really rare. We'll know in about 10 days."

Wait. And wait. And wait.

Ten days later, he called and told me to come back to the office. Fuck. OK, so I rented another car and drove up there again.

"We've got the results here," he said. "You actually do have a rare form of ovarian cancer."

"I what?" I was not believing my own ears.

He said, "Yeah. You have Stage 1 ovarian cancer." I did not know what that meant.

"Well, you're lucky because we got it early," he explained. "We're going to have to start aggressive chemo. Because we only found half the cell, that meant that it broke, and when ovarian cancer cells break, they flake apart and hide all over your body and multiply. That's why most women don't know they have ovarian cancer until Stage 3, and then usually it's too late because it has spread everywhere."

My first thought wasn't Oh, fuck, I'm going to die. My first thought was Okay, so what do we do to fix this? I wasn't in some gross state of self-pity or sadness. I was like, Let's get after this! I had done so much spiritual work in AA and that was such a help in being positive about the diagnosis.

My second thought was, Oh goodie! More surgery! More morphine! Once a drug addict, always a drug addict.

The doctor made an appointment for me with an oncologist, who would talk to me about the chemo and "get my port in." What's a port?

He explained it in terms I actually understood. "That's a little thing that we're going to put in your chest so we don't have to constantly stick needles in your arm to try and find blood. This way we stick the needle in the port and there's only one stick." Ah, OK.

A friend of mine named Chip drove me to Miami to see the oncologist. Dr. Longstead was the nicest doctor, an older gentleman who was so loving and kind. He showed me his treatment room and explained everything to me in such a nice way.

"Okay, we can get your port in next week," he said. "I'll set that up. Do you have any questions?" He paused a few seconds, and looked at me and sized me up. "I know this is hard."

Man, he made me feel so comfortable, so loved. I remember that feeling about him, hugging me like he was my grandpa. He was amazing.

Chip was literally on the edge of his seat out in the waiting room. "So what's up?" he asked. He seemed more nervous than I was.

"Not much," I replied.

We got in the car and I said, "Chip, I have cancer." The look on his face was something else.

Then we were quiet, just driving home. Two people in a car, one just diagnosed with cancer, the other one driving. Both being silent. I know we were both thinking about it, but I didn't want any of this shit to be awkward for anyone. It was the longest trip ever.

Finally I started talking—not about cancer—just about regular, mundane things. Just life as usual, no mention of that big fucking elephant riding along in the back seat.

The following week, my sister Elizabeth drove me up to Miami to get the port in. Bad me, I was looking forward to the morphine buzz and how it felt when I came out of it.

The doctor put the port in and all I could think was how weird it was to have this thing in my chest. It made me look like I had a third nipple so I called it my Triple Nipple. Being in AA taught me not to take myself too seriously, to laugh at my shit, laugh at myself, and don't sweat the fuckin' small stuff. Right now, this shit was out of my control, so there was no sense in making it worse by dumping more shit on it and causing more chaos. That's how I live today. If It's out of my control, it's not my monkey, not my circus!

So I got the port in and had to go see the Dr. H. in Boca again. He offered me the chance to do my chemo there, or said I could see an oncologist in Key West, thinking that might be easier for me.

"We'd love to have you here," he said. "But you figure out what you want to do."

I had a license, but I didn't have a car, so the decision kind of got made for me. Key West it was.

· 85 ·

St. Clay and The Hooker Sloth

Back at my apartment, I met an awesome new neighbor named Clay. One of the funniest people I ever met, very good-looking, great personality. Another gay guy, another Great Dane owner. What are the odds?

One day I was sitting on the stoop and as he was walking up the stairs to get around me, he cracked the funniest joke. I cracked one back, trying to one-up him. He did it right back, and went back and forth. It was completely hilarious. We were going to get along great.

I didn't tell him about my cancer diagnosis off the bat because I wasn't quite sure how it would land on him. On top of that, even though the doctors had given me that definite diagnosis, I wasn't quite sure whether it was really happening or not.

A few days later, I was sitting out on my stoop again, and Clay came out of his apartment.

"Hey! What's going on?" He was always so friendly.

"I don't know," I said. "Yeah, I do. I found out I got ovarian cancer."

Being the drama queen that he was, he was like, "Oh, my God. What do we do? What do we DO?" He wanted to control this and get up over it for me. There was another angel who came into my life.

Clay said, "I talked to people at my job who have been through this and they tell me support is Number One. So I'm going to come to every chemo with you, every doctor's appointment. You don't have to do this by yourself."

I was like, "Clay, you don't have to do that. I can handle it. It's just up the street. No big deal."

"No, nope, no way," he insisted. "When's your first appointment? I'm going to get a book. I'm going to get a nice pretty book. And then you're going to give me a list of all the stuff that you need and we're going to do this. I'm there, I'll take care of everything for you." You don't say no to Clay.

I went to the Key West oncology center, and had my first appointment with an Indian doctor (not the Native American kind, the east Indian kind). Clay went with me and he was more nervous than I was.

"I got stuff to do," I said. "Let's get this shit over with. I got weight to lose. I need to get back to work." My boss was actually great about it and told me to do whatever I needed to do. I was sure I could work while I was doing the chemo and take a vacation day if I really needed to. I had it all planned out... so did the universe, unfortunately.

The receptionist, who had very long black hair, looked like she just walked out of a Miami nightclub. She had the same snarky fucking attitude as Bon Qui Qui (a famous YouTuber... she had a big viral video... "I'ma cut you!")

She raised her gigantic false eyelashes to me and said, "Yes?"

"Hi, my name is Heather Gaines," I said, as politely as I could stand to. "I've got my first appointment here."

She smirked and was like, "Oh, I don't have you on this schedule." Very snippy and all, on her own little power trip.

"I made the appointment. It's supposed to be today," I said. My patience was already wearing out. She repeated that she couldn't find my appointment. "Oh, I'm sure you're here somewhere. Just take your seat." *Ugh.*

That girl was like 20 years old and she was trying to give me lip. This was not the kind, comforting office of the Boca doctor. I looked at Clay, and we both looked around at the people in different stages of hair loss and skin color. That's when it started to sink in for me, and I started to get a little nervous. After an hour wait, they called me in and Clay assured me he'd be waiting right there.

After a long walk down a twisty hallway, I landed in another waiting room for another twenty minutes. It was freezing fucking cold in there. It really sucks when you have to wait in those rooms because they might only have like *Tractor Illustrated* or something you would never want to read. You end up staring at the tongue depressors and the latex glove box. I was imagining what it would be like to blow up the gloves like balloons, and I knew I'd get in trouble if I start building log cabins with the tongue depressors, so I stayed still, just letting the doctor waste my time. He finally knocked and came in.

"Hi, I'm Dr. Sandarmakaran." No smile, no warm greeting, nothing warm about him.

"Hi." That was all I could muster.

He looked over my chart. I felt like I was just a big bother to him. I liked Dr. H. so much better.

"I guess we got a scheduled chemo for you. Do you have any questions?" *Really?*

"Well, you could be a little warmer," I said. I was just being honest.

"What?" He was really taken aback and looked at me with daggers.

I said, "I just, you know, would like to get to know my doctor a little bit."

And he was like, "Look, I don't have time for this." *Wow.*

I asked him if he could at least smile once in a while. He snapped back that if I wanted somebody to smile, I should pick another doctor. He added, "If you don't like me, I don't have to be your doctor."

WTF? No holds barred, I said, "Well, that is some bad bedside manner." *Fuck, is this how I'm supposed to start my goddamn chemo?*

"See the receptionist for your schedule and what you're going to have to do." He completely dismissed me and left the room.

"Okay. Thank you so much," I said, as he was closing the door behind him. Sarcasm has always been one of my strong points. HA!

His demeanor knocked me back and I felt nothing but sad. Clay was trying to be all upbeat and all I could think was what an asshole that doctor was and how I wanted to do this chemo somewhere else.

I went back out to the receptionist. I called her "The Hooker Sloth," moving so slow with her long fucking bright red nails and too-shiny black hair.

I said, "I need to book my next appointment." She said, "Fill out these papers and come back tomorrow."

I went back the next day without Clay. I was just dropping off papers, no need for a support person. There was a different receptionist, a woman named Shanna. She looked at the papers, looked at me, and at least she smiled. "I'll need a check for $10,000."

Cough, cough. Choke, choke, what?!

After I recovered from the initial shock, I realized that wouldn't be a problem because I had really good insurance. "My insurance covers this," I said.

She said, "It may, but in order to start your chemo, we need a check up front."

I fell back into shock and could barely speak. I said meekly, "But I don't have $10,000."

"Well, talk to your insurance," she said. "That's our standard procedure." I literally did not know what to say or do, so I said "thank you"—for what, I don't know—and left the office.

· 86 ·

MIRACLE ON 43ʳᴰ STREET

The next day at work, I tried to get some answers about the insurance from my boss, but could not. My co-workers couldn't believe it. I spent almost every day of the next month on the phone with supervisors at Blue Cross and got nowhere. I hope and pray you never have to fight with an insurance company to do what your premiums pay for. It is frustrating and maddening and exhausting.

It was about to the point where I was going to say *Fuck it, forget the chemo and I'll take my chances.* I make $9.50 an hour, how the hell can I pull $10,000 together? I decided to not think about it for the weekend.

I went to work on Monday and my co-worker showed me a coffee can with a label on it: "Heather's Cancer Fund." *GOD! Is this what it's come to?* Sandy said, so cheerfully, "I think this will help." I couldn't say anything else but "thank you." What a sweet thing to do.

One of the yacht owners (whose boat I washed) came up to the office and saw the can. He pointed at it and asked me that was all about. Most of my peeps at the marina knew about my diagnosis, but not about my money predicament.

I told him about the $10,000 fee, and that they wouldn't let me do chemo until I wrote them a check. He thought that was just plain crazy. We chatted for a few minutes, then he got what he needed from office and left.

About 30 minutes later, the guy came back and handed me a folded piece of paper.

"Here, this might help," he said. I unfolded it and realized it was a check. I hugged him and thanked him about four times. He smiled, turned around, and walked back down the dock.

I was so happy at the nice thing that man had just done for me. I looked at the check again and fell to my knees, bursting into beautiful tears. *That check was for $10,000!*

I pulled myself off the floor and ran down to his boat. I hugged him and his wife and said I would wash their boat for the rest of their lives. I would cater their parties. I would do anything, I was so grateful. They shushed me and said, "Heather, the only thing we want for you is to get better! So, go and start your chemo!" What amazing people live on this Earth.

The damn doctor got his check, but I still didn't understand what it was for, and I wanted someone to explain it to me. The practice manager told me it was in case there were "other costs," different drugs, etc. *Who knows what that meant?* She told me to go back to the horrible Hooker Sloth, who had another bunch of papers for me to deal with.

"What am I supposed to do with all this?" I asked. She told me to read through everything and be prepared for the chemo protocol.

"We'll schedule the day for chemo and you'll come in the day before for blood work. If your blood work is good, then we'll give you chemo," she said in her little snippy voice. "The day after that, they'll check to make sure your red and white blood cells are strong enough to protect your immune system."

I gave Clay all of these papers and he put them in a little binder. "Don't worry," he said. "I'll read all this stuff for you. You stay off the computer."

The whole thing just made me sad. Clay could see how down I was and suggested we go get some ice cream. I couldn't think of anything better. Ice cream solves all problems.

· 87 ·

GENTLEMEN, START YOUR DRIPS

The day before my first chemo, I went for my blood work (which was good) and so they told me to show up the following day at nine o'clock and they would start the chemo. Honestly, I didn't even know what it really was. I just knew I got my port in and they stick a needle there. *All right, I can handle that.*

Clay and I showed up five minutes early. Again, it was freezing in there. We walked into the "chemo room," which was filled with lots of big recliner chairs with poles next to them.

Where should I sit? I didn't know. Nobody told me. So I picked a chair next to a big, happy woman with glasses who loved to listen to country music. I named her "Country." She told me that she was on ChubbyChasers.com to meet a guy who was into overweight women. LOL!

The nurse came over and asked me if I was ready. *Ready for what?*

She said, "For me to put the needle in."

I asked, "In my arm?"

She said, "No, in your port." *Oh.*

She asked me why I didn't wear a zippered jacket or something. She said it was more comfortable to keep the IV in that way. I said, "Nobody told me, I didn't know what to expect."

She took a step back and said, "Didn't you go to the chemo class? Everybody is scheduled to go to a chemo class so you'll know what to expect during your chemo days and what to bring."

Mother fuckers dropped the ball on me again. Nobody told me about that. Well, fine, we'll just wing it.

She pulled my shirt down and told me she would count to three and put the needle in. I looked at Clay and he looked at me. 1, 2, 3.

"Oh, goddammit, that hurts," I said. I didn't expect that for some reason.

She said, "Oh, yeah, I should've numbed it a bit. Ha-ha." *Yeah, ha-ha. Story of my life.*

That first chemo was weird. The nurse explained that the first bag of liquid was something to coat my stomach so I wouldn't get sick. The second bag was steroids. Then the actual chemo, then Benadryl. Or something like that. So there were a lot of shit and poison because they told me it had to be aggressive.

To pump all of that stuff into me meant seven hours a day in the chemo chair, once every three weeks. *How hard can that be? No problem.*

That first time was uncomfortable because I was freezing and didn't bring anything to eat. The pillow was uncomfortable. The only good thing was that the chemo recliners were on the second floor, overlooking the Gulf of Mexico. The view was beautiful. I nicknamed it "Chemo by the Sea."

Looking out the window, I just daydreamed away. I did have a little puzzle book. Other people had all of their little creature comforts, little treats and such, DVD players, laptops. Next time I went I would look like I was camping there for a week.

Surprisingly, I felt really good for the next few days. The third day I was dead tired. I was told to expect that: the day after, you feel great. The next two days, you feel like shit, and I did.

Work was pretty easy to rearrange so that I could do the chemo and then recover. On my days off, I would get the chemo. I had some Mondays off so I could get the chemo on Friday and then I could work Saturday and have Sunday and Monday off. I never thought it was going to bother me much anyway. I felt fine because I was in good shape and had a good attitude. I was going to get through this shit with no problem!

A couple weeks after I went back to work, I was due for more blood work the day before my next chemo. Oops, bad blood work, no chemo! My white blood cells were way too low and my immune system was compromised. That's why I felt so tired. They told me to rest and come back in a week.

God, I was so bummed! That wrecked up my plan, which was six cycles of chemo and be done on June 1. Nice vacation here I come! But I learned early on in my sobriety that "projecting" into the future always got me in trouble and that I needed to stay in the present. Well, as we all know, I'm far from perfect!

· 88 ·

I Just Had Chemo, What's Your Excuse?

Part of the weekly bloodwork routine was to get weighed. If you remember, I was bulimic/anorexic, so the anxiety of getting on a scale to see if I had gained weight made that little demon inside rear its ugly head. I'd break out in a sweat just looking at that scale. A friend of mine told me she had gained 50 pounds when she was going through chemo. That petrified me. I wasn't afraid of dying; I was afraid of gaining weight.

I would close my eyes and wish, "Please do not say the number out loud, please do not say the number out loud" in hopes that I wouldn't be publicly humiliated. That meant I was fat, and that was enough to send me into a full-blown depression. Being depressed was definitely at odds with my decision to fight back and knock that cancer down. It was just a word to me, not a death sentence.

The doctors also instructed me to cut down on my exercising and eat more. Well, that was not going to happen. There were a few things that I was just not going to do.

I remember going out to run a mile, but I could only run maybe 20 yards. I was so tired and so out of breath, and I couldn't understand it. *Why was my brain doing this to me?* Well, it was the chemo that was doing it to me, but I was going to be that bad-ass who broke all the norms. The minute they told me I couldn't do it, I became determined to do it.

After my second chemo series, I went to work at my boat-washing job. After 30 minutes, I had to sit down. It actually took me three days to wash a boat that would usually take me two-and-a-half hours. That's when I knew shit was getting real.

The next round was coming up, with the bloodwork first, like always. My fingers were crossed and Clay and I were praying for lots of white cells. I just barely squeaked through, with just enough to allow me to take the chemo treatment the next day. Every treatment meant I was closer to the end, so I was ready!

We had learned over time that if you're going to sit through seven hours of chemo, you might as well be comfortable. So Clay had bags, and I had bags. Two pillows, two blankets, a cozy new workout outfit that zipped up, socks, slippers, candies, popcorn, coconut water, DVD player, laptop, iPod, magazines, and a book. I was not going to be uncomfortable if I was going to be in that chair for seven hours.

We were chatting with a few people, having a conversation that kind of reminded me of being in jail. "What are you in for?" The big difference was in the answer. Instead of "burglary" or "possession," it was "breast cancer" or "liver cancer."

People were in various stages of hair loss. I wasn't going to lose my hair because I was healthy. One of the things the chemo nurse told me was, "Heather, within 21 days of your first chemo, you're going to lose your hair." I looked at Clay and said, "No, I'm not." Every day I'd mark off the calendar: 10, 12, 13 days. No hair loss. *See?* I knew that if I really willed it, it wasn't going to happen. They just laughed at me.

Chemo gave me the weirdest sensations. I often didn't realize when they were changing the drip from the poison to the Benadryl or to the steroids. It was a huge concoction of a cocktail. I remember being in the middle of a conversation when the drip switched to Benadryl and I passed out in the middle of a sentence. When I woke up, I started talking again, thinking that I was still having that same conversation. Clay was like, "Heather, that was like an hour and a half ago." He thought it was so funny to watch me pass out in mid-sentence.

Chemo can definitely make you do irrational things. There was this awesome white watch I saw online, a Casio G-Shock. I had no idea that I ordered it. No idea. Imagine my surprise when I got this package from Amazon and it was the white watch I'd always wanted. *Who sent me this? Did you send me this? How did somebody know that I really wanted this watch?* I thought maybe Amy did and just didn't want to tell me, but nope. The chemo made me do it!

When I saw my credit card bill with a charge for $300 on it, I knew I had ordered it, and I sent it back. Another time I called a friend and said, "You know what? I haven't been to Spain in a long time and I was just looking at tickets. Let's go to Spain next weekend." That sounds like the kind of stuff I would have done when I was drinking, but I was stone-cold sober—just all chemo-ed up.

After the last chemo, I really felt okay, just super-tired. Seventeen days had gone by and I still hadn't lost my hair. I was just so ecstatic that I was going to prove them all wrong.

In the interest of trying to keep my love life alive, I made arrangements to finally meet Geoff, the guy I'd been talking to online and on the phone. It was so nice to meet him and be out of my "cancer life" for a few days. We made plans to meet again the following weekend, which we did.

Sunday morning I woke up to find my curly hair all over his bed. It was Day 20. They were right. *Oh, God, my HAIR.*

"What's that?" asked Geoff, staring at my pillow. He looked pretty horrified.

I was like, "Oh, it's nothing." Honestly, it didn't bother me after that initial shock. The first thing I was going to do when I got home was cut my hair short and make it all cute and spiky.

That lasted about a week before it started getting very, very thin. *Time to order a couple of wigs.* My perception of myself was so based on the physical things: my body, my hair.

One thing for sure was that I was never going to be that girl with the crooked weave. You see a lot of people with their wigs a little askew, and other people look at them and say, "Oh, look, that poor girl has to wear a wig." The other thing I would not do is wear one of those turbans wrapped around my head because I didn't want people pointing at me and going, "She has cancer," and looking at me all sad. That was not going to happen either.

So after the short hair started falling out, I asked my friend to shave off the rest. After four concussions and a fractured skull, my head must have been pretty horrific-looking; the fracture from the fall down the stairs in Mexico left a Star-of-David-shaped scar. I thought I was going to have the ugliest bald head in the world.

It was not! My head shape was pretty good. It took some getting used to—I can't say it didn't. Let's look at the good side of losing my hair: I didn't have to shave my legs or my bikini area. The other side is that I lost my eyebrows and had no eyelashes. That kind of got to me, but I fixed it with makeup and eyeliner. I made sure that I kept my head tanned so I wouldn't look sickly, and wore cute little baseball caps. That's how I got through that part of the chemo.

Geoff was so nice about it. The next time I went up to visit him, he was like, "Oh, my God, you're so beautiful!" It was nice to have somebody that I could visit because it made me feel sort of normal, even though my life was far from it in those days.

· 89 ·

Double Your Chemo, Double Your Pain

The next couple of attempts at getting chemo failed because my blood work was not good. Twice, my cell count was so low I had to have a blood transfusion. I was getting sicker, but I wasn't throwing up like some people do. In a crazy way, I was actually looking forward to throwing up so I could lose the weight I so was obsessed with.

My salt content was *waaay* low. Potassium deficiency. The doctors were like "Heather, you have to stop exercising because you're losing salt." People would see me and my big ol' bald head walking whenever I could: on the beach, around town, wherever. "I said, "I can't eat salt. Salt will give me cellulite." That physical-body thing, you know.

My doctor was hilarious. One day he got his prescription pad out and wrote, "Two bags of potato chips" on it. "If I prescribe it, you have to do it," he said. I took him up on it. *Jesus, those chips were so, so good.*

Six months went by and I was having a hard time. I'd only like gotten through three, maybe four of the chemos because my body was ignoring the treatment, like rejecting it. I don't know whether it was the low white-cell count that was knocking me on my ass or what.

Not long after that, they called me into the doctor's office and said, "So, Heather. Unfortunately, the chemo isn't working." I looked at Clay. *What do you mean it's not working?*

"We're going to have to double the poison and we're gonna see you every three weeks. These will be eight-hour sessions instead of seven."

The "chemo life" made me fucking crazy, and I thought I was about to be done with it. Now they're telling me I have to do another fucking six to eight months of this shit. *Okay. All right. Whatever we got to do, whatever we got to do.*

Not being able to work became a worry, but we are very fortunate in Key West because there are a couple of organizations here that help people in the service industry if you are sick, can't work and can't pay your bills.

A non-profit called The Sister Season Fund was so helpful to me and I'm very grateful for them. I had to fill out a ton of paperwork and do all this stuff, but they paid my rent for the whole time I did chemo. (Rent is not cheap here.) Another non-profit, the Cancer Foundation of the Florida Keys paid my utilities. These people were angels, in big contrast to the increasingly shitty chemo. I was getting more and more tired. Chemo was just kicking my ass.

For the next round, they decided on a different protocol. Instead of the two-day ritual of bloodwork/maybe-chemo, now it was going to be bloodwork-chemo-Neulasta. *What's Neulasta?*

It's a horrific shot that's supposed to feed your bone marrow and make more white blood cells. If you need Neulasta, it means the chemo is not attacking your body the way it should. For 36 hours after the shot, you feel awful. Horrible. Every inch of my body was in just horrible pain.

I didn't believe them when they warned me about it because, well, I have a very high pain tolerance. Well, I am here to tell you, that shit was no joke! I felt like I was being tasered. They gave me all kinds of pain pills, everything you could imagine. Nothing touched it. All I could do was lay in bed and pray to God, like, "I know you can't take this pain away, but maybe, maybe you could just lessen it for an hour this time?"

The weirdest thing was that it seemed like every time I had to go through that, a *Lord of the Rings* marathon was on TV. The music and the colors of *Lord of the Rings* were very soothing to me for some reason.

During the new chemo regimen, my best friend Amy came down to see me for a week. She couldn't believe how sick I was. I wasn't like throw-up sick, but I couldn't eat and I had no strength. I just hurt.

She told me later on that she thought I was dying. She always tried to come into my room with the biggest smile and ask what she could do, or try and make me laugh. Then I would fall asleep, and she would go sit on my front porch and cry. Amy and Clay became very, very close friends.

One of the worst parts was when my vision started getting blurry. It's fine now, but then my eyes hurt so bad after chemo that I finally had to see an eye doctor. She explained that the chemo was messing with my eyes because it was attacking my whole body. As my body changed, she had to keep giving me different prescriptions for my contacts. On one of eye exams, she moved her finger from right to left and my eye wasn't following it.

She wanted to send me to an eye institute in Miami, and so Elizabeth drove me up there. My appointment wasn't until eleven o'clock, so we decided to check out a perfume store in a nearby strip mall first.

We tested a bunch of fragrances and had a nice little time. Around 10:30 we walked out and across the parking lot, just chatting away. We didn't hear the F-150 truck, and he evidently didn't see us, and so the next thing you know we were literally flying through the air after being hit by an F-150 truck. Elizabeth went sailing off to the left and I spun and landed on my back, both of us unconscious.

When I came to, there were all kinds of people around us, and they were like, "Where's your shoe?" *Why do they gotta know where my shoe is?* The pavement was scorching because it was like 100 degrees that day.

Somebody asked, "Do you know where you are?" and no, I did not. I asked what happened and a man told me we had been hit by a truck. I started laughing and looked up at the sky. *God, for real? Really? What else you got for me?*

A woman's voice said, "This girl's going through cancer. She needs help." I was asking about my sister. I heard her say, "I'm over here." I asked Elizabeth if she was okay and she said she didn't know.

An ambulance showed up about five minutes later and took us to the hospital. Luckily, no broken bones, but lots of bruising. I damaged my tailbone because I fell on my bony ass. I was in the hospital for a couple of days because I think I got another concussion and they were worried because my white blood cells were so fucking compromised. I was having a hard time breathing. So there I was, out of work for another two weeks.

I remember my coworker calling me, saying, "Heather, you have to come to work tomorrow." I was like, "Dude, I can barely sit up."

She was like, "Well, I heard somebody say that if you don't show up tomorrow, you're going to be fired."

What the fuck? I'm a great employee. I've got to deal with chemo and now I've been fucking run over by a truck and they're gonna fucking fire me?

I called my boss to ask what the hell was up. "Yeah, I'm not supposed to say anything about this," he said. I didn't have a choice, I had to go to work and it was horrible. I could barely bend over to tie a boat up. *But you know what? I did it. I did it because I had to.*

It was a trick to try and work while I was having all of the side effects, not to mention being hit by a truck. Late in the day I was doing my paperwork and all of a sudden I got the most screaming pain in my head. I thought I was having an aneurysm. *My God, do I have a brain tumor?* Something was happening. It was the most excruciating pain. Back at my house there was a prescription for pain meds, but I kept them at home, never thinking I would need them at work.

A friend coincidentally stopped by to say hello and saw me all wrenched up in pain. I just kept screaming that something was wrong with my head and to please help me. *Call Clay, Clay!*

Clay dropped what he was doing and hauled ass to the marina. The look on his face when he saw me was so pitiful. He was worried, but he was trying not to cry and be there for me.

"Everybody out!" he yelled, scooted everyone out of the office, and shut the door. "Here's your pill, Heather, here, hurry, take the pill." Clay just cradled me and rocked me back and forth until the pain subsided. God bless Clay.

I called the doctor because I didn't know what the fuck was going on. He explained that bad migraines can be par for the course for some chemo patients. I was like, "Someone could've of fucking told me that. I thought I was dying. I thought I had a brain tumor or something." That was one of the scariest, scariest things.

Well, chemo was my life and I had to deal with it. I'd go to work and come home; that's about all I could do. I was determined to try and work the last four months even though I couldn't do a whole lot of anything. I was still going to my AA meetings, where sometimes I would just rage a bunch of nonsense just being so pissed off about the chemo and all of that pain. But it was such a loving group there and no one was saying, "Oh, shut up." They were all just very empathetic and compassionate. Without them and Clay, I don't know what I would have done.

———

HEATHER FEATHER

Here is something Clay wrote about me. He was the wacky neighbor in the sitcom of my life. He was the Ethel Mertz to my Lucy Ricardo, the Ed Norton to my Ralph Cramden, the Shirley to my Laverne.

He lived two doors from me, and he burst into my life just like the best friends you see on TV. Ours was a friendship borne of proximity, but nurtured through time. He made me laugh, made me worry— but also inspired me. I taught him how to persist through pain and he taught me how to be a friend. In 2009, that friendship would change everything, and his lessons would need to be relearned again and again.

Here is Clay's story about me. It's called, "Heather Feather."

Just like on all the other months of Fridays that Heather was scheduled for chemotherapy, I called her to confirm the time of her appointment.

Heather said, laughing, "It's always at ten o'clock on Friday mornings."

"I know," I said. "I just like you to remind me." I smiled to myself as I hung up the phone, standing at the desk in my bedroom. I thought about the past year of Heather's chemotherapy. It had been a long journey, starting in January right after she was diagnosed with Stage 1 ovarian cancer. When she told me about the doctor's diagnosis, I said immediately, "I'm in! Whatever you need."

So, *we* began treatment. It's funny, now that I think about it, that I say "we" when I talk about her diagnosis and treatment. It's just that throughout the past year, we'd become a team. I was the coach. She was the player. *Did I just make a sports analogy?*

I wanted Heather to focus on getting well—winning, if you will. I was in charge of reading the boring cancer pamphlets, keeping her distracted in the waiting room and making sure the prescriptions got picked up. Heather was in charge of staying alive.

While taking a shower that Friday morning, I thought about how different this year turned out to be from what we expected when we first talked about her treatment. We were told it would be six weeks of chemo, every Friday, for about one to three hours. I think it was called "big chemo" and "little chemo." Then there would be an evaluation of her progress.

There was no reason to believe we wouldn't be finished with the chemotherapy by the beginning of summer. Heather was already making plans for her vacation.

"Great," she said. "Maybe I could lose a couple of pounds before I go to St. John's!"

"Atta girl," I replied. "Keep your eye on the prize."

But we would soon learn that cancer rarely follows a schedule, and it allows absolutely no time for a summer vacation.

Later that Friday morning while getting dressed to go to our appointment, I wondered when she realized that the chemo wasn't working. I think it was sometime in the late spring. Part of the treatment plan was a weekly test of her white-cell count. The nurses wanted to be sure that her body was strong enough to sustain the impact of the chemo. Heather's numbers were always on the lower side of acceptable, so they were constantly testing.

As the weeks passed, her numbers fell at an alarming speed. Soon, she was too weak for her regularly scheduled appointment, so she would have to wait a week for her white blood cell count to come back up. The next week, the numbers would be down again. It was like being up for parole every week, waiting to see if you are going to get out or be denied.

Heather and I were sitting in my living room some months into the treatment, watching some horrible movie on Netflix. Heather's taste in movies is the same as a 13-year old boy: blockbusters with lots of car chases and explosions. I, on the other hand, have the attention span of a gnat and was focused solely on the popcorn.

I asked Heather if she had thought about the cancer support group the clinic told her about.

"Yeah," she said. "But isn't that for people with cancer?" Quite the smarty-pants.

"Well, yes, I guess," I replied. "But wouldn't that include you?" I mumbled, shoveling mountains of popcorn into my mouth.

"But I mean, it's for people who really have cancer," Heather said.

Well, after spitting out bits of popcorn and laughing uncontrollably, I threw the remote control at her. She finally looked away from the movie, grinned and said, "What? The rollercoaster of cancer is that it goes up and down."

There was a time she collapsed at work and called me from her office. The pain was excruciating. Her head was pounding. Could I please bring her meds? Heather was crying. I had never heard her cry before. And for the first time through all of this, I was truly scared. *I* was scared!

Using my spare key to her apartment, I grabbed her medication and drove as fast as I could to her office. I was saying over and over, out loud as I drove through red lights, blew through stop signs, and passed every car in my way, "Hold on, Heather. I'm coming. Hold on. Hold on."

When I got to her office, she was rocking herself in her chair. For a second, I froze at the door when I saw her. She looked so small and frail, very much like a person with cancer.

My heart broke. I told myself, Keep it together, Clay. And then I took over, cleared the office and locked the door. When I held her there in my arms, the floodgates of her tears opened up. I said to her, "It's okay, I'm here." I rubbed her hairless head where the pain was the worst. We sat quietly while we waited for the pain pills to kick in. Heather dried her tears and started to feel her pain passing. She mentioned how good the air-conditioning felt when it kicked on.

She was finally able to stand up and we were both slightly embarrassed by the intimacy of the crisis. "You'll do anything to try and have sex with me," I kidded. Seeing that I'm gay, that was pretty funny. We both laughed. It was going to be okay. The rollercoaster went up; the rollercoaster went down.

There were unscheduled blood transfusions (two) and more medications all through what turned into a more than a year of chemo. Never once did she question it; she did what she had to do, despite the fact that the weekend following her Friday chemo was always brutal. She never complained. She never gave up.

"Tell me what you want me to do and I'll do it," Heather said to her doctor one day. I could tell she was growing impatient with the process. We were already months past the original "we're done" date. I knew she was thinking it, but didn't dare say it out loud: *Why wasn't the chemo working? Why? Why were we still coming here?*

We tried to pretend it was no big deal when the doctor added on more appointments, extending our finish date. Just a schedule change. No biggie. We were both afraid that if we said what we were thinking out loud, it might jinx things and make it true.

The routine for the Friday morning chemo appointments was always the same. I arrived at the doctor's office 50 minutes before she did. I wanted to make sure everything was set before she got there. No surprises.

I would greet Tina, the receptionist (perhaps better known as The Hooker Sloth), and wondered who she was banging on her lunch hour. She always came to work dressed like she was auditioning for a dance show on Telemundo. Did we really need to see her thong while waiting for our appointment?

While we waited, I always made a mental note of who was wearing a wig and who was not. Weeks before losing it, hair was *the* one thing Heather kept mentioning she feared.

I remember that when the chemo nurse, Janice, told us about the side effects, what to expect and when to expect it. She pinpointed on the calendar—almost to the day—when Heather could expect to lose her hair. Ten minutes later, driving home on our scooters, Heather yelled to me across the lanes on the boulevard.

"Well, at least I'm not going to lose my hair," she said, with all kinds of fake confidence.

I almost crashed my scooter. "What the hell are you talking about, you bonehead? Janice just told you when you're going to lose your hair."

"When did she say that?" Heather asked, just as if she never heard a word Janice said. I didn't know if she was kidding or in some extreme kind of denial.

"Heather?? Ten minutes ago. What's wrong with you?" I yelled over my shoulder.

The cars were honking because the light had changed. We both laughed.

In time, Heather embraced her beautiful bald head. She even had a bumper sticker on her scooter that read, *I'm too sexy for my hair.* It was true. Heather has a beautiful head! Who knew?

The following Friday, I was back at the doctor's, waiting for Heather to arrive. I pulled out the old magazines I had donated to the reception room and surveyed the snacks I'd brought for the long day ahead. It could be anywhere from six to eight hours; we never knew.

I had pretzels with peanut butter for me, new gossip magazines for Heather, and candy for the nurses. Heather arrived with her pillow and blanket, her unstoppable energy, and more snacks and magazines. We were loaded and ready to go. She looked tired to me, but I didn't mention it.

Sometimes we were in a private room. Sometimes, like this particular day, we were in the community room. The nurses always made a place for me, and I was grateful for their kindness. The room had seven chairs with bags of chemo attached to long metal poles next to each chair. Heather had settled into the chair while Janice attached the chemo to the plastic port that had been inserted into Heather's chest.

That part always made me flinch. I tried to keep myself and Heather distracted by making fun of the sports bra she was wearing. I looked around the room and realized that except for Janice, the nurse and me, everyone was bald. I pretended not to notice.

I said "hey" to the other patients while they were being hooked up to the machines. They had watched Heather and me, and wondered if we were a couple. They wondered if I had cancer. I wondered if I'd brought enough pretzels with peanut butter for everybody.

The morning progressed and Heather's sedatives were beginning to kick in. She was talking loudly and not making a lot of sense. I made a mental note to make fun of her later (lol). She began to drift off to sleep, and I'd check to make sure she was warm and comfortable. Janice checked the vitals of her patients and then she and I talked about Key West real estate, her new grandchild, and an upcoming cancer benefit.

She played '70s rock and classic country music on the CD player in the room. I knew every tune and Janice and I sang along while she did her work. I read *People* magazine while the Eagles sang "Peaceful Easy Feeling." There's a line in there that says, "I know you won't let me down." It seemed awfully appropriate.

The community room was a cross-section of patients. Different cancers, different backgrounds, different stages, one disease. I sat in one of the treatment chairs and joined in on the polite conversation the other patients were having. The weather, the kids. Fishing in the Keys, the tunes that always filled that room. The conversation deepened as to why we were all there. What kind of cancer do you have? When were you diagnosed? What are your symptoms? How is your insurance? What's your treatment plan? Do you want pretzels with peanut butter?

Pretty soon it was just me and an older guy talking. His name was Ross. He was probably in his 60s, but looked much older. I wondered if his darkened skin color was from the sun or the radiation. I learned that he was married and he and his wife owned a house on Sandstone Street. I told him I used to live on that street back in the 1990s, and we both smiled at how small Key West was. I learned that he had colon cancer and he was in Stage Four. Stage Five is his death. He looked to me like someone who was dying. I kept my poker face on throughout our conversation; no surprise reactions, no look that reflected the voice inside my head that was shocked or worried or sad. In fact, I showed very little reaction to anything I saw there.

When you see so many people hooked up to machines, fighting to stay alive for such a long period, it becomes kind of normal. The conversation about what happened in the bathroom or who died over the weekend had become part of our weekly visits. Nothing was too personal for us. We no longer had time to be appropriate. The clock was ticking in that room and we all heard it. Ross got a call from his wife while we were talking, and I could tell she asked what he wanted after his treatment. He laughed and said, "Vodka!"

"Right on, brother," I said, and gave him a wink.

"She's great," Ross said after he hung up. "But she gets tired. We've been fighting this thing for three fucking years." He trailed off, but I sensed he had more to say.

"The bills are crazy, man," he added. I thought he might have gone to sleep. "Thank God we have the house."

I nodded, and he continued. "I don't know," he said. "They keep telling me it's working, but every month it's more bad news."

I stared at him, and we made eye contact. He went on. "They just found it in another place in my body. It keeps spreading." It was just Ross talking. The rest of the patients were either listening or falling asleep from their medication. Janice was working on her paperwork over in the nurse's station in the corner.

After a minute, Ross said to me, "You know what, Clay? Eighty percent of the people with my diagnosis die from what I have." I looked at him, and then I looked at the floor.

"Then that means twenty percent live, right?" I said. "I remember reading about surviving cancer, and one of the points they made was not to get lost in the statistics. You're a person, not a number. And maybe the strategy should be not to accept being part of the 80 percent, but to focus on being in the 20 percent."

I continued. "Look, Ross, I can't begin to understand what you're going through, but I watch Heather and I see her fighting this thing. I can't help but wonder if I would have the same kind of strength she has if I were in her shoes. I hope so. But the one thing I do know for sure is that Heather made a decision after her diagnosis that she wasn't going to give up, that this cancer thing would not come to define her. It would be something she endured, but it would not be who she is. And that knowledge seems to be what pulls her through each day. She is a person, not a statistic."

Ross was quiet, but stared straight into me. I suddenly remembered where I was and I felt embarrassed and exposed. I felt that maybe, as I often do, I said too much. I looked over at Heather and realized that sometime during my conversation with Ross, she had opened her eyes and started listening. When I caught her eye, she smiled at me and I smiled back.

The day was almost over. The bags of chemo had been changed with the passing of the hours. Several of the other patients had left and some had just come in. Then the elderly woman who sat two chairs over suddenly stood up and said, "Okiedokie Smokey." Then she left. She hadn't said a word all day.

Heather and I could barely stop laughing. Ross and I were trading restaurant war stories about being bartenders back in the day. We laughed at all the horrific things we'd done to rude customers and discovered that we both served a lot of cocktails that had a little "something extra" in them.

I was the kind of the bartender who walked to the table munching on one of the customer's French fries while carrying the plate to the table. "Who gets the fries?" I'd ask, dripping with enough sarcasm to serve as ketchup.

The stories got more and more outrageous as Heather joined in with stories of her own chef adventures. The others in the room were laughing so loudly at our stories that the head nurse came in and playfully told the room to keep it down.

Sometime during the conversation, she and Ross started sharing their cancer stories. She was talking about what she planned to do after she was done with chemotherapy. People with cancer don't usually talk about the future. But then again, Heather doesn't do anything the usual way. I was proud of her as I sat back and listened to her talk. I thought about how lucky I was to be sitting next to her. There are moments in our lives that are filled with grace and that was one of them.

In some ways, none of us were strangers in that room. Whether we knew each other's names was not important. We were all fighting the same thing, on the same battlefield. We knew some of us would make it and some of us would not. There were already patients we no longer saw just in the course of 10 months. Where did they go? Were they OK? Sometimes we asked; sometimes we didn't want to know.

All the laughter died down as the final bags of chemo were finished around the room. Ross got another call from his wife who said she was on her way to pick him up. One by one, Janice unhooked the machines from each patient's ports. I folded up Heather's blanket and packed up her bag. She scheduled what we hoped would be her last deployment for chemo. She'd have two months off to recover, and then she would return to the doctor to learn whether she needed more.

I saw Ross out of the corner of my eye as he was leaving. He shook my hand and said, "Hey, Clay, it was good to meet you, man." And then unexpectedly, he gave me a hug.

Heather and I headed out on our scooters. The sun had begun to set here and the street was filling up with traffic coming onto the island. The sky was painted with colors and the air felt warm.

It had been a long day and I asked Heather how she was feeling. "I'm tired," she said. I wonder if she meant she was tired from the day, or tired from the last year. She let out a sigh as we stood in the parking lot. There wasn't much more to say. "Let's go home," I said. "Let's go." And we literally rode off into the sunset.

A note about Clay...

Clay, rest his soul. He was bipolar and couldn't quite get hold of it. The meds never were quite right for him. It sucked because as tortured as he was inside, I couldn't help him. It seems the funnier the person, the more secretly depressed they are. Clay had attempted suicide before, in 2014 or 2015. If it weren't so serious, it would have been funny. We joked about it anyway. It was a comedy of errors.

After my treatment was over, he kind of wandered off into a different life; he started writing and got in with a new group of literary friends. He tried to overdose himself on pills, but it didn't work and he was pissed off that he was still alive. There he was, totally out of it from the pills, and he decided to wander a couple of blocks from his house to the pawn shop in an effort to buy a gun. He was so fucked up he couldn't even fill out the paperwork.

After that, he was totally frustrated. There was one of those two-story chain hotel across the street from his house, so he got the idea to go over there in the middle of the night and make his way up to the roof. He jumped, landing feet first, shattering every bone in both feet. That didn't kill him, either.

Clay reached out to me about a month after that and told me everything. He was completely depressed because he hadn't been successful, and now he had all of these bills for doctors, hospitals, surgeries, etc. I was happy I could be there for him after all he did for me.

I called his mom (we had met once—I was the "crazy cancer neighbor") to see if she could provide him with some financial help because he was so worried about all the medical debt. Two months later she called to tell me that Clay was dead. Somehow he had gotten a gun and shot himself in the head. Well, I guess it took that time!

That was in 2016. I miss my dear, funny friend.

· 90 ·

All Clear

After a year and a half of the aggressive chemo, after CT scans and PET scans and bone scans and whatever, they told me it looked clear. It looked clear!!! That was one of the happiest days of my life and I was floating on air. For real!!

By then, a lot of people knew my cancer story and knew that I could help people who had been diagnosed or had a friend or relative who had been diagnosed. People would get in touch and ask me questions and I would be supportive. When you first get that diagnosis, you are scared and in the dark; I got that. I was happy to help anybody wade through that bullshit. I would go back to the chemo place every once in a while to drop off a bag of organic suckers for the patients there, just to lift their spirits because I knew what it was like.

People always ask me how I survived it, and I always tell them I did it with a little sense of denial, a big sense of humor, and a REAL big positive attitude! I never once sat in my little apartment and thought I was going to die. There were a lot of times I wish I could have died because I was in so much pain, but I never quit fighting it.

I had this awesome faith that it wasn't going to kill me. People would sometimes say, "This too, shall pass." Well, if you know me, don't ever say that to me because fuck that, you all don't know what 36 hours of Neulasta is like. That was one of the hardest things I had to suffer through.

Looking back, I think I was lucky. I don't think the cancer would have been found if I hadn't stopped drinking. I wouldn't have gone to a doctor about my belly growing; I would have just told myself I was getting fat. If I had still been drinking and gotten diagnosed, I wouldn't have gone to the doctor anyway. So with the love of a lot of people, I made it.

It took a while for my hair to grow back. When it first started coming back in, it was like bleached-white. Oh, my God, people are going to think I'm an old-ass. What an ego! So I went and had it shaved again, believe it or not. I had been bald for so long I had kind of gotten used to it. You know, I actually got asked out on many dates with my bald head—that was amazing!

After I got the "all clear," Geoff and I went up to Miami to go shopping and celebrate. We went to Neiman Marcus and got the big popovers they're so famous for. Yummy and decadent! Not long after that, I met Geoff up at Disneyworld to go on the rollercoaster extravaganza.

My relationship with Geoff endured while the chemo was happening, but not without our ups and downs, a few lies, and some PTSD thrown in. Once I had to bail him out of the psych ward after an "incident." Geoff was retired Navy and retired Army, very military. He had served in Afghanistan. He had a lot of intimacy issues, and I'm not talking sex—I'm talking about being able to relate to another person on a just-relax level. There were lot of red flags with him. He was another one who kind of broke my heart, but not as bad as the others. I'll leave it at that, but I will say that the "blue-eye candy" sure was nice while it lasted.

· 91 ·

THE RIPPLE EFFECT

As of 2020, I have been nine years cancer-free and 13 years sober. My core is back to being strong and that has created a ripple effect of positivity in my life.

One of the greatest things I get to do is to talk to people who've been diagnosed and help them. I love putting chemo kits together for people. If I know someone's going to start chemo, I can give them a list of things they'll need or I'll even send them all the stuff. Maybe I should call it Heather's Chemo Kit? There's an idea!

I also work with a lot of women who are trying to get sober and get off drugs. When I was three months out of chemo, I met a great lady who is a marketing person for most of the hotels and cool places in Key West. She invited me to a paddleboard demo down at the beach. That was something I'd never done.

So I went down there with my bald head and my cute little daisy bikini, and I got on that paddleboard. It changed my life. I felt like I was actually walking on water! Oh, my God, I need to do this. Where can I do this? My friend told me about Lazy Dog (my current employer)—a paddleboard and kayak company, owned by my boss, friend, and mentor, Sue Cooper.

I start doing some race training at Lazy Dog and went to my first race in Pompano Beach. It almost killed me! After hanging out with this super-energetic paddleboarding group, Sue asked me if I might want to work at Lazy Dog. Um... no brainer. Awesome!

I had been washing boats at the marina for about six years, and I loved it. It was a good gig, but it seemed like the administrative end of things was kind of falling apart. There were some bad politics between some of the people there. I'd be all happy and come to work in a place where everyone was so negative, which is not for me.

You know, I wake up every morning. I say my prayers and I get ready to grab my day. I don't wake up saying, Oh, fuck, I gotta get up. Some days are harder than others, but most of the time I get up with a positive attitude.

So I gave my two-week notice at the marina and started my new Lazy Dog life in 2012. That first race I placed in my age group, which was pretty crazy. It opened a whole new world of friends and interests for me. I get to travel a lot for the races, and I'm finding a new tribe after being "tribeless" for years. I feel so fortunate to have these awesome people around me all the time.

Not that I don't still have the occasional terrifying adventures. After being at Lazy Dog for a few years, I got invited to go to Hawaii, which is my co-workers' favorite place. They go to Holly's (a condo on the ocean), in Kauai every year to do Na Pali, a 17-mile paddleboard race down the coast.

They said, "Oh, Heather, it's gonna change your life. You're gonna think of everything from your childhood; all your happy memories will flash before your eyes. It's going to be the most beautiful race ever."

I almost died on that race! You have to paddle off the beach and make a blind, hard left and haul ass so you don't run up on the reef. The waves are huge because it's downwind. I wasn't used to that – we don't have waves in Key West. Bouncing up and down like that made me feel like my bladder was going to drop out. I'd fall, and my paddle would go one way, my hat would go over there, and I'd be scrambling.

Paddling and paddling, and man, was I so seasick! I was in a paddleboard race and I was throwing up and couldn't stop. I dropped to my knees to rest a little and get some water. Back to paddling, going up and down. I felt like I'd only gone three miles.

Sue told me about a time she got dehydrated when she was racing. She stopped for a while and recovered. Was that it, was I dehydrated? Maybe I'll just lay down on my board for a minute and take a little nap. Uh-oh, that's a red flag. You can't do that because you're in the ocean. You could fall off and there are sharks, you know. Don't want to be Shark Lunch.

Every time I stood up, I'd feel sick. I'm just going to maybe sit here for a while and wait for a support boat. I sat there for a long time in the hot sun and then I saw a red Zodiac dinghy heading my way. It was just like the Old Spice commercial where the hot guy, his hair blowing in the wind, pulled right up to me. I was so dehydrated, I didn't know what was real and what wasn't. I was actually hallucinating.

"Are you okay?" asked the Hot Dinghy Guy. I was pretty focused on him and said, "Are you real?" Anyone who is thinking they can take a nap on a paddleboard and is asking people if they are real is not quite with it.

"Of course, I'm real! But you're not feeling good, right?" he asked. Right.

He gave me some Gatorade. I started feeling better right away. Then I learned that I only had three miles left to go in the race. I had gone a lot further than I thought I did. Oh, my God, really, I had already gone 14 miles?

"About 25 yards from here, it's going to flatten all out. It's a piece of cake the rest of the way," he said.

"I'm going to finish," I declared. I have never quit a race in my life. Hot Dinghy Guy asked me again if I was okay, and I assured him that I was.

I remember getting to that finish line, which was also situated on the biggest drop-off at the beach. I caught a wave that pummeled my ass and threw me on the beach. But I finished. I will add that I will never, ever, ever do that race again, no, no, no.

"You'll think about your childhood… it will be such a beautiful race…" HA! It was the survival of the fittest for me, no joy ride. A couple of years later that opportunity came around again and I turned it down. Sue said, "How about if it was a relay?" Hmmm. And so I did the relay, and have done it four times now!

My life is constantly changing, and always for the better. I wake up every morning with a great attitude and try to carry it through my whole day. As you know, I'm a big believer of the concept of "move a muscle, change a thought." If you're having a shitty thought or are in a shitty head space, go for a run, go for a walk, go for a swim. Give in to your urge to submerge. Jump in the water. Dive deep. Let that water roll off your back. The endorphins will explode and make you feel nothing but good.

These days, I'm always looking for the next challenge, the next adventure. Last year, I did a crazy thing called "Everesting," as in Mount Everest. That's where you have to climb the equivalent elevation of Mt. Everest (that's 29,029 feet, y'all) in 36 hours.

Jesse Itzler, who is another one of my mentors, rented a snow basin in Utah. You had to hike 1,750 feet straight up, 17 laps. That is some crazy elevation, and for somebody from Key West, the altitude was a real factor.

I trained my ass off for four months. I made eight laps before I couldn't breathe because of the altitude. My oxygen level got extremely low, so they had to pull me out, but that was okay because I climbed 18,510 feet in 18 hours. I'll be going back to do it again this summer because I have to get a red bib. That means you've completed the challenge. I want that bib.

Yep, I still take risks and love adventure, but now I take on challenges with a clear head and sheer determination, instead of being dangerously impulsive and doing things just for the sake of filling that "big empty hole." I finally came to understand that I was out of control because I was out of control—my parents didn't teach any of us kids how to function in the world because they didn't know how themselves. It wasn't their fault… they did the best they could because they had their own limitations.

I came to terms with my mother's death by learning to understand that she would want me to live my best life. I know she is always with me; she actually comes to me in my dreams.

And those men I allowed to treat me so badly? I got over that by learning how to love and respect myself, and I was able to forgive them by acknowledging that they were sick as well.

I learned that being of service to others feeds your soul, lifts your spirit, and makes you a more empathetic person. For so many years, I was missing all of that; no wonder I felt like a shell.

Once you understand these things, it sets you free. I'm never, ever, ever going back.

Some days I look at my old mugshot from when I was arrested in the Keys. It's there to remind me to remain where I am now: no sad-clown masks, no pretending.

I'm just Heather, and I AM FREE.

EPILOGUE

WHERE TO GET HELP

Alcoholics Anonymous
aa.org
Hotline: 1-800-8391686

Alcohol.org
alcohol.org
Hotline: 1-866-484-1712

SAMSHA (Substance Abuse & Mental Health Services Administration)
samsha.gov
Hotline: 1-800-662-HELP (4357)

THEN AND NOW

Unless you're one of those people who reads the end of the story first, congratulations! You've just completed your ride on Heather's Death-Defying Rollercoaster! You might be amazed I'm still here and standing (I am), sober (yep), happy (yep) and healthy (hella healthy). But do you remember how we started this whole thing: "Am I dead yet?"

Sometimes you have to come full fucking circle to see where you've really been, so the answer to that question is, yes. The Heather who doubted herself, never felt good enough, never fit in, and drank and drugged her way through half of her adult life is dead. The Heather who took crazy risks, craved attention and love, and hurt people she cared about along the way is dead. And I couldn't be happier.

THEN

When I used to think about what an alcoholic was, what came to mind was a dirty, unshaven man in a trench coat, lying in the gutter. I thought, "How could I be an alcoholic? I don't even own a trenchcoat!" I wasn't like that. I just liked the feeling of uninhibitedness that drinking gave me. But the more I drank, the harder it was to get that same feeling. It wasn't until I got sober that I realized alcohol is a depressant. It had stopped working for me, so what did I do? I brought in its evil twin, cocaine. Cocaine made it easier to drink, even though that feeling I was searching for never returned. I couldn't live without either one. I lost control of everything...and didn't care. Check yourself and really take inventory of how much you're really drinking, and don't lie to yourself.

Being a slave to alcohol and drugs was my job, my breath, my lifeline. I had two thoughts: "If I don't get a drink, I'm going to die" and "If I continue drinking, I'm going to die." Back and forth, back and forth, pushing me further into that black tornado drain. Don't lose sight of yourself; be aware.

Looking back on all of that insane behavior, I used to tell myself I was just having fun and being crazy. I felt invincible and indestructible (you know, "ten feet tall and bulletproof"). Youthful drinking in my teenage and early adult years—that's all fun and games in your twenties. When you're still doing that stupid shit in your thirties, it's a problem. And then into your forties? Come on. Time to take a hard look in the mirror and grow up.

There were many times I could've died. I must've had (maybe still have?) a guardian angel looking out for me. That poor angel. Probably said a bunch of four-letter words that angels shouldn't say, looking after my ass. Everybody has their angel. Be grateful for her and listen to her when you feel that devil tapping you on the other shoulder.

NOW

When I first got sober, my sponsor asked me a few questions, namely, "What changes do you hope to see in sobriety?" My answer was simple but profound, and I wrote it down in a journal I was keeping at the time:

I hope to feel whole again, and to be at peace with myself.

I hope to be able to look in the mirror and feel good about myself, physically and spiritually.

I hope to do something about my emotional intimacy, maybe have a date.

I hope to reinstate my license.

I've done all those things, and more. You can, too.

Here's the thing: Once I became sober, I saw how wasteful my life had been, and I experienced overwhelming feelings of regret and guilt (the "ick"). I learned that my self-centeredness and dishonesty stemmed largely from my drinking and drugging, and I drank because I am an alcoholic. Now I can see how even my most distasteful past experiences can turn into GOLD. I now share those experiences to help my fellow alcoholics and addicts, particularly newly sober peeps. They say reaching out my hand to another person who is struggling will help me stay sober, and I believe that.

I learned that the people I thought were my friends weren't really my friends. That happens a lot with alcoholics—the only thing you have in common with the people you used to hang out with is the bond of drugs and alcohol. As the booze and drugs wore off and that black tornado lifted, my circle of friends got real small.

Understand about H.A.L.T.: Hungry, Angry, Lonely, Tired. I frequently check in with myself to see which one of those things I'm feeling and then adjust my sails ("Check myself before I wreck myself!"). I have to let my ego go and practice humility. I ask myself, "Do I want to be right, or do I want to be happy?" I've learned to pick my battles!

Get out of your own way, have an open mind and a little bit of willingness. Have you ever stayed up all through the night, and right before the sun comes up it's super dark outside? A huge part of my life was lived in that place right before the dawn, full of the blackest darkness and without any hope. Stay out of your "shitty diaper," Find your tribe. Stay where your feet are, move a muscle, change a thought! If you want it, earn it.

Whenever you get down on yourself, just remember this line from Auntie Mame: "Life's a banquet, and most poor suckers are starving to death!"

Don't starve yourself! Treat yourself and the people you love with kindness and respect, be good to yourself, and spread that good around you. You can do this. You can have peace and be whole again. Just set out to do it!

Today? My life isn't perfect, but it's pretty damn awesome. I've learned to love myself and trust myself more. I've learned to not take myself too seriously. I still have some insecurities, like when I look in the mirror and a distorted body image looks back. When that happens, I've got good, solid tools to deal with it. I ask, "What's going on in my life right now? What's making me see something different in the mirror?"

I find joy by feeling grateful that I get another shot at this amazing life. I find joy in my crazy, adventuresome friends. I love my job, paddleboarding, adventure, and adrenalin (big surprise there!). I live my life by staying in the present and trying not to project into the future. I look for the positive in any situation and always look for ways to spread joy...and hope.

If you're reading this and you're struggling, and your life seems out of control, I want to give you hope. And listen to me: there is always hope.

Let my words and my experiences and my life now be a beacon of hope to you. I want to let you guys know that anything is possible as long as you get out of your own goddamn way. Even though you might be in that darkness now, that dawn is coming and man, it is bright.

Know peace.
Know God.
No peace.
No God.

HEATHER'S DESIGN FOR LIVING

Start your day with gratitude.

If you can look up, you can get up!

Move a muscle, change a thought.

Don't let your mind quit before your body does—you always have about 40% left in the tank!

If you want to have it, you've got to earn it.

Live in the solution.

Be selfless.

Stay out of your head; it's a dangerous place to live.

Believe in something greater than yourself.

Leave your ego at the door—your ego is not your amigo!

Talk to yourself like you would your best friend.

Don't let anyone tell you no.

It's never as bad as your head tells you it is.

There's a light at the end of the tunnel...and it's not a fucking train.

STAY AWESOME.

WHATEVER HAPPENED TO...

Hey, you didn't think I'd leave you hanging, did you? I can't just tell you my life story and then make you wonder what happened to everyone, right?

Heather is nine years cancer-free, living her best life in the Florida Keys, working at Lazy Dog as a SUP instructor, tour guide, and PaddleFit instructor. She is still sober, works out like a fiend, and has amazing legs for an almost-60-year-old. Still looking for love—but this time, in all the right places. Would love to share her experiences and humor at your next conference or retreat (hit her up at HeatherGainesSpeaks@gmail.com), but don't be surprised if she shows up in a mini-dress and drops a few F-bombs!

Richard (Buff) died of lung cancer.

Chris died in prison at the age of 49 after being convicted on manslaughter and a firearms charge.

Eric (Dink) is married with two children. He recently became a new grandpa.

Elizabeth has a daughter and lives not too far from me.

Amy still lives in Virginia Beach with her husband, and is still my best friend. She has two grown sons.

Andy is living a great sober life. He married a wonderful woman and lives in St. Thomas in a beautiful home that overlooks the ocean.

Mark seems to have disappeared into the ocean mist, never to be heard from again.

Jamie is a chef in Florida, working on a boat that's seen better days. Still owes me a fucking plane ticket.

Captain Kent keeps a home in Florida and travels the world as a yacht captain.

Dale passed away in 2008, not long after he watched his alma mater win the national college football championship. He was only 54.

Clay very sadly committed suicide in 2016. He was bipolar and had attempted to kill himself several times prior. God rest his soul.

Acknowledgements

I'm eternally grateful to the Divine, to all the great things in spirit, and to all those here on Earth who help me in this life.

I am grateful beyond words for my blood family, both past and present—y'all will never know how much I love and cherish you.

I also want to thank my best friend, Amy, who witnessed so much of the stuff in the book, who loved me then and still loves me unconditionally today. Amy, you have seen me at my ultimate worst and again at my best. You're my forever cheerleader. You get me! Thank you for praying for me always!

I can never be grateful enough for my boss, mentor and above-all friend, Sue Cooper, who for the last nine years has heard story after story and finally pulled the trigger for me to write this book. When I met you, I never could have imagined how my life would change for the better. Thank you for your creativity, your appetite for adventure, and for teaching me to say YES! Thank you for believing in me!

Special thanks to the great Jesse Itzler (who I met through Sue). Your workouts and the BYLR pushed me to believe in myself, to be more confident, and to know that I always have "40% left" when I want to quit.

A heart full of gratitude to Master Chief Tommy Taylor (Ret.), who knew me when I had no self-esteem and no confidence, and who made me feel like I belonged and was worthy. The P.T. Raiders taught me to challenge myself and push me to my limits. Tommy, you are my HERO.

None of this would have been possible without my AA posse, who helped me find a new design for living, and helped this phoenix rise from her ashes. And to Vidal: thank you for your spiritual guidance. I wouldn't be where I am today without it.

Special thanks to Stan and Dana Day, and Kurt and Marianne Winters for believing in my project, and to all of my awesome Kickstarter backers who literally made this book possible! I will always be grateful to each and every one of you.

Finally, to Jenny, my Managing Editor, and LeAnn, my Development Editor and Designer: thank you for walking me through this process and being right by my side the entire way. We did it!

———◦∞◦———